MS and Your Feelings

⌘ ⌘ ⌘

[A] long overdue book on managing the emotional impact of MS! *MS and Your Feelings* addresses specific psychological challenges and provides in-depth questionnaires and practical strategies to help you understand and ultimately meet those challenges. … [R]eaders will undoubtedly recognize themselves and their emotional challenges, and consequently, feel validated and less alone.

— Christine Ratliff, editor, *MSFocus*
The Multiple Sclerosis Foundation

Finally a book that takes an honest look at what someone is feeling as they live with a chronic illness. Shadday's insight and direction for exploring those unspoken feelings is an immediate help by offering tools to recognize and communicate our feelings to others. After reading *MS and Your Feelings*, I felt better about myself with a deeper understanding of why I feel the way I do. Everyone close to me will be receiving a copy of this helpful book.

— Kathleen Wilson, MFA, MA
Founding president & CEO, *MSWorld*

In *MS and Your Feelings*, Allison Shadday gives us tools that can change our perception of MS and of ourselves as MS patients. The simple exercises she recommends can empower us to amend the way we respond to the presence of MS in our lives. Allison's words might ultimately enable us to view MS as an ally in our journey toward self fulfillment rather than as an enemy to be fought every step of the way. Allison has done a great job and a great service to MSers.

— Judith Lynn Nichols, author of *Women Living with MS*
and *Living Beyond MS: A Women's Guide*

DEDICATION

⌘ ⌘ ⌘

For all those who face great challenges
with great courage.

Ordering

Trade bookstores in the U.S. and Canada please contact:

Publishers Group West
1700 Fourth Street, Berkeley CA 94710
Phone: (800) 788-3123   Fax: (800) 351-5073

Hunter House books are available at bulk discounts for textbook course adoptions; to qualifying community, health-care, and government organizations; and for special promotions and fund-raising. For details please contact:

Special Sales Department
Hunter House Inc., PO Box 2914, Alameda CA 94501-0914
Phone: (510) 865-5282   Fax: (510) 865-4295
E-mail: ordering@hunterhouse.com

Individuals can order our books from most bookstores, by calling
(800) 266-5592, or from our website at **www.hunterhouse.com**

Project Credits

Cover Design Brian Dittmar Graphic Design
Book Production Hunter House
Developmental Editor Kelley Blewster
Copy Editor Nancy Faass, MSW
Proofreader John David Marion
Indexer Candace Hyatt
Acquisitions Editor Jeanne Brondino
Editor Alexandra Mummery
Senior Marketing Associate Reina Santana
Customer Service Manager Christina Sverdrup
Order Fulfillment Washul Lakdhon
Administrator Theresa Nelson
Computer Support Peter Eichelberger
Publisher Kiran S. Rana

MS and Your Feelings

Feelings

HANDLING THE UPS AND DOWNS OF
MULTIPLE SCLEROSIS

Allison Shadday, LCSW

Hunter House
PUBLISHERS

Text reprinted from *The Six Pillars of Self-Esteem* by Nathaniel Branden, copyright © 1994 by Nathaniel Branden. Used by permission of Bantam Books, a division of Random House, Inc.

"Back" copyright 2005 by Estate of Jane Kenyon, Reprinted from Collected Poems with permission of Graywolf Press, Saint Paul, Minnesota.

Library of Congress Cataloging-in-Publication Data

Shadday, Allison.
MS and your feelings : handling the ups and downs of multiple sclerosis /
Allison Shadday. — 1st ed.
p. cm.
Includes index.
ISBN-13: 978-0-89793-489-3 (pbk.)
ISBN-10: 0-89793-489-X (pbk.)
1. Multiple sclerosis—Popular works. 2. Multiple sclerosis—Psychological
aspects. I. Title.
RC377.S53 2007
616.8'34—dc22   2006033937

Printed and bound by Sheridan Books, Ann Arbor, Michigan
Manufactured in the United States of America

9 8 7 6 5   First Edition   11 12 13 14 15

Contents

⌘ ⌘ ⌘

List of Journal Exercises

These are indicated in the text with **

Foreword

⌘ ⌘ ⌘

Multiple sclerosis (MS) is an inflammatory, degenerative disease of the brain and spinal cord that, if left untreated, will produce major physical disability in 50 percent of patients within 10 years, in 75 percent of patients within 20 years, and in approximately 90 percent of patients within 25 years of their diagnosis. Since MS may first manifest itself in people in their late teens to mid-30s, even patients with a more "benign" course may experience significant disability by their mid 40s to mid 50s, a time in life when most people experience their most productive and fulfilling years.

MS is not uncommon. In North America its prevalence is estimated at 1 in 700 to 1,000 people.

Fortunately, the outlook for patients with MS has significantly improved with the introduction of new therapeutic agents that modify MS disease activity, including Type I Beta-interferon (Avonex, Betaseron, and Rebif), glatarimer acetate (Copaxone), Tysabri, and mitoxantrone (a chemotherapy drug often used to treat certain types of cancer). These medications reduce relapse rates, reduce disease activity as seen on magnetic resonance brain scans (MRI), and, in some cases, reduce risk of future disability. Other medications, such as cyclophosphamides, azathioprine (two immunosuppressive drugs), methotrexate (a cancer treatment that interferes with the production of DNA), and high-dose steroids may also improve disease control and long-term outlook. Collectively, these and future medications act to control and correct the abnormal biological processes causing the disease.

A second category of therapy addresses the symptoms of MS. In addition to the well-known problems of weakness, loss of vision, impaired speech, and impaired balance and walking, there are pervasive and often under-emphasized symptoms of increased fatigue, as well as cognitive disturbances such difficulties with memory, concentration, and multi-tasking. Significant depression is experienced by the large majority of patients with MS at some time in the course of their disease. Spasticity, difficulties with bladder control and recurrent urinary tract infections, impaired sexual function, and various pain syndromes are common consequences of MS. Fortunately, effective therapies are available for these important symptoms, but, all too often, patients are not adequately treated because the doctor doesn't ask, and the patient doesn't tell, perhaps at times out of embarrassment, which results in an incomplete treatment plan.

It is important for patients to keep a list of symptoms and concerns and to be certain that the doctor addresses each of them, explains the basis of the symptoms when possible, and provides a treatment plan for each symptom. Thus, depression, if present, must be identified and treated with medication and supportive psychotherapy, and the causes of bladder dysfunction should be accurately identified and treated. Physical and occupational therapy must be employed to improve strength, coordination, dexterity, and walking, and it must be supplemented by medication to reduce spasticity. Behavioral strategies must be employed to conserve energy, reduce fatigue, and to reduce the impact of cognitive difficulties.

As newer medications reduce the risk of developing severe or progressive disability, more MS patients can anticipate longer, more active, and more productive lives. This prospect greatly magnifies the importance of recognizing and treating the symptoms produced by MS, rather than just focusing upon the biological abnormalities that cause the disease, in order to maximize patient benefit.

A third pathway of therapy must be devoted to protecting the inner person, and it is this critical task to which this book is devoted. We must enable a person with MS to come to terms with the impact of MS upon their self-image and sense of self-worth, to develop or improve psychological coping mechanisms for real or perceived changes in their life status, and to promote changes in the way they are perceived and treated by significant people in their life.

- ❖ How does a person with MS cope if they "look really good," but have difficulty with memory and excessive fatigue?

- ❖ How can they respond to the unspoken criticism of unsympathetic or imperceptive coworkers or employers?

- ❖ How does a person with MS avoid emotional isolation or the emotional impact of physical isolation?

- ❖ What type of emotional support will most benefit someone with MS?

- ❖ How can someone with MS develop these critical insights, and who will help them in this quest?

This book is a response to these questions. Every person with MS may benefit from the valuable advice Allison Shadday provides on coming to terms with and understanding the emotional impact of discovering they have MS, coping with the fear of the future, and prevailing over the adverse impact of negative emotions. She advises and exhorts the person with MS to summon the energy and the resources necessary to overcome depression and maintain self-esteem. Following Allison Shadday's advice may help a person with MS find and use the weapons necessary for a proactive response to MS, rather than remain a passive victim, and instead be an active seeker of solutions, without which response no medical or therapeutic program will be fully successful.

Learning the lessons and incorporating the insights offered in this book should be empowering and will place a person with MS at the helm, in charge of directing their future. A person with MS who reads this book learns that they are a member of a community with shared challenges, shared fears, shared disappointments, and with shared successes, particularly in the way they exhibit courage and determination and preserve dignity. Allison Shadday writes about MS in language that rings true to a person with MS, in ways that may assist each person in finding their way to a better self-understanding about their relationship to their unwelcome companion.

In this book, Allison Shadday combines thoughtfulness, intelligence, and wit with her practical experience as a clinical social worker, who has devoted her career to assisting fellow MS patients. The result is this very valuable book, which should be read by all people who have MS. When they are finished reading it, they should give it to their family members, lovers, doctors, nurses, therapists, and probably to the staff members of the human resources office where they work. This very important knowledge can go a very long way toward helping a great many good people.

— Dr. Stanley Cohan, M.D., Ph.D.
Medical Director, Providence Multiple Sclerosis Center

Acknowledgments

⌘ ⌘ ⌘

From the moment this book was conceived, I was surrounded by a community of people who carried me through the process of completing it. I am deeply grateful to everyone who helped make this project possible.

I am fortunate to be associated with a publisher who feels a passion for helping others. Thank you, Kiran Rana, for giving this book all the time and attention it needed. Thank you, Jeanne Brondino, for having faith in the book from the get-go. Thank you, Alexandra Mummery and Kelley Blewster, for being kind and gentle and honest as you edited. Thank you, copy editor Nancy Faass, for your attention to detail. Thank you, Christina Sverdrup and Reina Santana, for helping to get this book into the hands of those who need it.

Thank you, Dr. Stanley Cohan, for giving of your time, expertise, and most of all your compassion.

Thank you, Marie Schwab, Kay Hartley, Renate Rose, Gina Mattioda, Sue Schindele, Stephanie Swanson, Chris Ratcliff, and Dr. Linda Miller, for your input, suggestions, and unique perspectives.

Thank you, Susan Wingate, for sharing your enthusiasm and commitment to writing.

Thank you to all of those living with MS who have given generously of your time, thoughts, and feelings.

Thank you, Sven, for being a supportive, loving, and encouraging husband. You are my rock.

Thank you, Mom and Dad, for never giving up on me.

Above all, thank you to my clients who inspired me to write this book. May your strength, courage, and determination give others the same.

Important Note

The material in this book is intended to provide a review of information regarding the emotional impact of multiple sclerosis. Every effort has been made to provide accurate and dependable information. The contents of this book have been compiled through professional research and in consultation with medical and mental-health professionals. However, health-care professionals have differing opinions, and advances in medical and scientific research are made very quickly, so some of the information may become outdated.

Therefore, the publisher, authors, and editors, as well as the professionals quoted in the book, cannot be held responsible for any error, omission, or dated material. The authors and publisher assume no responsibility for any outcome of applying the information in this book in a program of self-care or under the care of a licensed practitioner. If you have questions concerning your nutrition or diet, or about the application of the information described in this book, consult a qualified health-care professional.

All the names and occupations used throughout this book have been changed to protect confidentiality.

Introduction:
Understanding Is Everything

For years I lived in denial. Despite my disturbing symptoms— chronic pain, blurred vision, disorienting dizziness, staggering numbness, and debilitating fatigue—I pretended I was fine because to do otherwise meant that something was seriously wrong. However, as a medical social worker, I suspected that my physical ailments might be early signs of multiple sclerosis.

A little bit of knowledge is a dangerous thing. Working primarily with those in advanced stages of the disease, I knew what the worst-case prognosis looked like. Each day I provided support for my homebound clients as they struggled to deal with the effects of MS. During our visits, I held their hands and offered words of comfort while they grieved their losses and fought to find quality in the lives they now lived. I saw clients lose their ability to work, walk, and worse. Meanwhile, I foolishly clung to the magical belief that my professional role could shield me from illness. But each time I felt a part of my own body go numb or my vision go haywire, I knew that their present might be my future and it terrified me.

The day finally came when my husband and I decided to start a family and I had to face my fears directly. Before we had a child, I needed to get to the bottom of my health problems.

With a sense of dread in my heart and a knot in my stomach, I went to see a neurologist and scheduled an MRI—a helpful MS diagnostic tool. When the doctor slapped the MRI films up on the light box and pointed to the numerous lesions on my brain, I instantly recognized the telltale signs. He confirmed what I instinctively knew. I had multiple sclerosis.

Suddenly, every defense I'd concocted over the years slipped away. The thumping sound of blood pounded in my ears. My breath stopped and I felt faint. I imagined my future and it looked bleak. With tears pooling in my eyes, desperate for some shred of reassurance, I asked my doctor, "How am I going to cope with this?" His reply was pathetically inadequate and cold, "I don't know... take Valium?" I had never felt more hopeless or alone.

But I'm *not* alone. Someone is newly diagnosed with MS every hour of every day. Unfortunately, this is a chronic, unpredictable, progressive, neurological disorder that generally strikes early in life. At least two million people worldwide have the disease. Including family members, MS has an impact on about six million people. In the United States alone it is estimated that 400,000 people live with this disease—almost half a million people.

Tragically, few MS patients and family members are ever offered the emotional support they need to cope with this insidious, life-altering illness. (There is a saying, "Think globally; act locally.") To meet this need in my own community, I started a private counseling practice to help other patients overcome the emotional turmoil caused by chronic illness. This work has drawn on both my personal and professional experience.

After providing support for hundreds of MS clients, I began to notice more clearly a pattern in the challenging psychological symptoms that crop up in reaction to the disease. These symptoms include anxiety, low self-esteem, isolation, relationship conflicts, sexual dysfunction, grief, and depression. Often, the emotional consequences of MS can be more debilitating than its physical symptoms. However, with supportive counseling and education, those with MS can learn to manage the painful feelings associated with the disease and maintain a high quality of life, despite the physical disabilities that may develop.

Unfortunately, due to many obstacles, including financial constraints, mobility problems, transportation issues, and a lack of qualified mental-health providers, the majority of MS patients never receive the professional counseling they need.

That's why I wrote this book. My desire is to reach the hundreds of thousands of patients and family members who are looking for ways to cope with the day-to-day challenges of this disease. Now, patients with questions about managing the emotional impact of MS can find many of the answers they are looking for right at their fingertips, while flipping through these pages.

MS and Your Feelings is the first book written for all those looking for comfort, direction, and strength, while facing the emotional ups and downs caused by this devastating disease. Throughout the book you will hear personal stories of other MS patients and how they have managed to overcome the inevitable emotional obstacles MS presents. As you learn about how others have dealt with their emotions, you'll find the inspiration and motivation needed to handle your own. By using the insight-oriented exercises provided in these pages, you'll learn more about your personal psychological reactions to the disease and uncover meaningful ways to begin healing both emotionally and physically. These exercises are meant to be shared with loved ones, in the hope that they may also gain a deeper understanding of the role MS plays in your lives and how its effects may be minimized. The professional guidance in this book comes from someone who not only counsels others, but who also contends with the disease. I truly understand what it is like to live with MS and its challenges and my wish is to provide you with the validation, reassurance, and coping skills that can help you survive and thrive with this disease.

How to Use This Book

Since the focus of this book is on managing the emotional impact of MS, each chapter addresses specific psychological challenges and how to meet them. Although we all experience the disease of MS differently, these chapters represent some of the most common and yet complex issues that patients and their families struggle with. This book can also be shared with family, friends, and health-care professionals to help them gain a greater understanding of the difficulties you face due to this disease. If you're seeing a counselor or if you decide to see one in the future, I would encourage you to have them read this book as well. The information can help them establish a foundation of background on MS and provide them with a context about your illness and the emotional consequences that can arise from living with the disease.

As you begin reading, you may want to start with the chapters that target problems you're dealing with currently. The book is structured so that you can skip around from chapter to chapter.

Chapter 1 addresses the difficulties and advantages of obtaining an accurate diagnosis of MS. Patients discuss what it is like to first hear that they have MS and share their responses to the initial diagnosis. The benefits of finding the right doctor and treatment options are also addressed. Common MS symptoms are reviewed and the reader is encouraged to begin monitoring their own specific symptoms.

Chapter 2 explores the various psychological responses patients have to the initial diagnosis. Patients and families are asked to respond to an MS diagnosis questionnaire to begin facilitating the adjustment process and to open up the lines of communication among family members. Suggestions are offered to help patients reach a point of disease acceptance so that they may begin to take proactive steps toward managing all aspects of the disease.

Chapter 3 discusses the importance of recognizing and acknowledging one's inner feelings and helps readers identify how their emotions impact their physical symptoms. You are encouraged to identify your coping style and strengths. Another questionnaire is used to explore how MS is impacting your life.

Chapter 4 examines some of the typical emotional responses to MS including fear, loneliness, anger, guilt, and sadness. Patients share their experiences of how they worked through these feelings. Specific strategies are offered to deal with each of these issues.

Chapter 5 explains why depression is so prevalent among MS patients. Over 50 percent of us will suffer from a depressive episode during the course of our disease. Signs and symptoms of depression are discussed and stories of healing are shared. Approaches to treatment and guidelines for selecting an appropriate counselor are also offered.

Chapter 6 illustrates the connection between stress and MS symptoms. Several stress-management techniques are provided and explained. Readers are encouraged to identify their personal stress triggers, using a 60-day symptom log, as well as a stress journal exercise.

Chapter 7 validates the challenges MS poses to maintaining healthy self-esteem. Several self-esteem building exercises are offered and readers are shown how they can find new ways of defining themselves and their self-worth. Readers are encouraged to identify their unique gifts and talents.

Chapter 8 recognizes the many losses we experience during the course of this illness and helps readers recognize the various stages and types of grief. The importance of recognizing our losses is emphasized and many easy-to-follow suggestions are given to help you move through the grief process and on toward hope. A grief questionnaire is used to help you better understand your own reactions to loss.

Chapter 9 confirms the huge role fatigue plays in the lives of most MS patients. Types, symptoms, and causes of fatigue are explained. The reader is asked to rate their own fatigue triggers and several successful strategies for managing fatigue are recommended. Patients tell their stories of coping with exhaustion. Families are given tips on how to support the patient in minimizing fatigue, as well.

Chapter 10 explains the challenges to communication that MS creates, and case examples are used to show how miscommunication commonly occurs. The reader is given a quiz to evaluate their own communication style and several suggestions on how to improve both speaking and listening skills are offered. A final section on talking to your kids about MS is included.

Chapter 11 stresses the importance of maintaining relationships and enhancing intimacy with your partner. Patients give examples of how the support of others has gotten them through the toughest of times. Tips for increasing your social network are offered and the value of MS support groups is considered. The causes of sexual dysfunction are explored, as are creative solutions to common problems with intimacy.

Chapter 12 deals with the cognitive challenges that many of us experience. Types of cognitive symptoms are explained and facts and myths about cognitive impairments are discussed. Several compensatory techniques are offered to help reduce the impact of cognitive dysfunction.

Chapter 13 gives family members a chance to honestly and openly voice their feelings and experiences of MS. This chapter explores how the family is impacted by the disease, and several loved ones share how they cope with MS.

Chapter 14 leaves the reader with some positive thoughts about living with MS.

In the Appendix, Dr. Stanley Cohan discusses the medical advances that are being made in the fight against MS and tells us what we can hope for in terms of future treatments.

The resource section provides an additional wealth of information regarding Internet sources and further reading for those who want to learn more.

The reader questionnaires are an integral part of this book. I urge you take the time to write out your answers. My clients have always gained the most benefit from these exercises when they actually put pen to paper. This allows you to go back and reflect on your responses and also see how your responses change over time. Another great advantage to writing down your thoughts is that you can then share them with your loved ones and begin to process your feelings about your responses together. These conversations can be rich with insights and "aha" moments and can further your understanding of each other's experiences. I would encourage you to buy yourself a journal dedicated to use in conjunction with the exercises in this book, and use it solely for this purpose from the get-go. Your journal can be as simple as a yellow-paged notebook.

Finally, this book is based on witnessing hundreds of people who have found ways to overcome the many emotional and physical hurdles that MS has put in their path. My clients have been my greatest teachers. So, with the best of intentions and hope for your future, I share with you these lessons that I've learned. May they help make the ups and downs of your life with MS a little easier.

chapter
one

Knowledge Is Power:
Getting an Accurate Diagnosis

*The most effective way to ensure the value of the future
is to confront the present courageously and
constructively. For the future is born out of and made
by the present.*

— *Rollo May,* Man's Search for Himself

By choosing to read this book, you've accepted the challenge of confronting the present and you're taking an active role in constructively shaping your future. If you're currently living with MS, you've experienced firsthand how terrifying it can be to hear the words, "You have multiple sclerosis." An MS diagnosis can strike panic in the bravest of souls. It changes your life forever.

As someone who lives with the disease, I understand how the news can turn your world upside down. All your previous assumptions and expectations are replaced with uncertainty. It can literally feel like the beginning of the end. But it is possible to move beyond the initial reaction of fear and panic and eventually to integrate the illness into your life. Over the years, I've watched with amazement and admiration, as hundreds of my clients have made peace with the disease in their own unique ways. Listening with an open heart and a curious mind, I've seen patients resolve their emotional

8

conflicts with grace, dignity, and determination. Their courage has inspired me to write this book. Although identifying details have been changed to protect their privacy, many of these clients' stories are shared throughout the chapters.

Each person navigates the course of their disease differently; yet, the first step for all of us is to get an accurate diagnosis. For a number of reasons this can often be an extremely difficult undertaking. Some of you may be in the process of getting diagnosed—others may have been given a nondefinitive diagnosis. I encourage you to read on and get the facts, in order to proactively take part in the diagnostic process. Otherwise, you may be discounted or left lost in limbo with a misdiagnosis.

Defining MS

THE MYSTERY ILLNESS

In order to fully participate in the diagnostic process, it helps to know some of the basics about the physical aspects of MS. In many regards, MS is still a mystery. We do not yet know what causes it or why it affects some people and not others. And, although we now have drugs that can help treat MS, we still don't know how to cure it. That said, we have learned a great deal about the disease since it was first described by the French neurologist Jean Charcot in 1868.

Put simply, MS is a disease of the central nervous system that involves the brain and spinal cord. The central nervous system controls all our bodily functions and movements. Needless to say, the healthy functioning of this system is critical to our ability to think, feel, and move.

The brain sends and receives signals and the spinal cord uses a network of nerves to transmit those signals to different parts of the body. Our nerves are coated by a type of insulation called myelin. Problems occur when disease activity triggered by MS causes the protective myelin to break down and replaces it with scar tissue.

This process is called demyelination, which impedes the flow of signals from the central nervous system to the body. For example, while your brain may be trying to tell your legs to move, they may not be getting the message. So, damage to the nervous system can result in difficulty with day-to-day functioning. We will talk more about the specific symptoms associated with MS later in this chapter.

MISSING SIGNALS

The nervous system can be compared to the electrical system that powers your home. Nerves are somewhat like electrical wires and the myelin sheath is like the protective plastic coating on an electrical wire. The process of demyelination is often compared to stripping away the plastic coating on an electrical wire, compromising the wire. The myelin sheath, which protects and insulates the nerves, is gradually destroyed by the disease process of MS.

When this occurs, the nerves (axons) are no longer able to effectively do their job—which is to quickly communicate and send messages easily from brain to body. This means that once the damage has occurred, the information must travel in a less efficient route and push through less direct channels. Depending on the location and number of lesions, the brain's ability to communicate can be greatly disrupted.

Imagine driving into the mountains, only to be sent on a detour because a mountain pass is closed. It takes you hours longer, driving through snow and darkness, to get to your destination, and you're exhausted at the end of the trip. This is the effect that demyelination can have on your ability to function and on your energy level. In MS, this decrease in the brain's ability to process information is a primary cause of profound physical and mental fatigue. Your brain has to work much harder to get its messages across. Hence, you can become tired just from thinking.

MS is considered an autoimmune disease of the nervous system. The word "multiple," in multiple sclerosis, indicates the many areas of demyelination from repeated attacks that occur over time. The word "sclerosis" refers to the scarring that appears on the brain and spinal cord. We don't know why, but this process of demyelination differs vastly from patient to patient, and, hence, the course of the disease also varies widely. You simply can't predict how the disease will affect you. Often symptoms will resolve and patients will regain function after an attack, or some residual damage may remain, but they experience a partial recovery.

Possible Causes

by Dr. Stanley Cohan

There is also some evidence to suggest that viral infection may be the initiating step in most, if not all, cases of MS. There is a critical need to prove, or disprove, the pivotal role of viral infection in causing MS. If viral infection is the initiating event, treatment with antiviral medications could prevent onset, or rapidly terminate the disease process in its earliest stages, before significant damage to the nervous system could occur.

Environmental factors, including air, water, and food-borne toxins, temperature, sunlight exposure, and nutritional deficiencies, as causes or contributors to the risk of acquiring MS, all have their adherents. Some of these proposed environmental contributors to MS risk are potentially significant, yet little or no valid scientific evidence exists to support these possible causes. Rather than dismiss these theories as invalid for lack of corroborating scientific evidence, well-designed scientific studies should be performed on the more biologically plausible of these theories, in order to establish or eliminate them as important possible contributors to MS.

Although MS is not a hereditary disease in the traditional sense (you don't inherit MS), genes may play an important role in determining why one person exposed to a virus, which could cause MS, contracts the disease, while another person, exposed to the same virus does not develop MS. Although some candidate genes have been identified, the picture is currently incomplete. With proper identification of MS-risk genes, it may be possible to develop medications that turn off

(cont'd.)

these genes, or block the biological effects of proteins produced by these genes, thus turning off the disease process once it has started, or preventing the disease from ever starting in a genetically susceptible individual.

TYPES OF MS

The medical community has attempted to categorize the different types of MS and the following are the currently accepted categories:

- ❖ Relapsing remitting MS is a condition developed by about 20–30 percent of patients and is characterized by periods of relapse, followed by periods of full or partial recovery and remission.

- ❖ Secondary-progressive MS is developed by about 50 percent of patients with Relapsing Remitting MS—typically 10 to 20 years after their initial diagnosis. This type of MS is characterized by a slow increase in disability without remission.

- ❖ Primary-progressive MS is developed by only about 12 percent of patients. This condition causes a slow, but steady, increase in disability from the onset of diagnosis.

- ❖ Chronic-progressive MS occurs in another 10–20 percent of patients. This condition involves a slow worsening of symptoms, without periods of remission, but the onset is much slower than that of Primary-Progressive MS.

As Dr. Cohan mentioned in his Foreword, most MS specialists feel hopeful that as more patients benefit from the new disease modifying treatments now available, we will see less disability and a reduction in the number of cases that become Secondary-Progressive. We will talk more about how these treatments, and other medications, can benefit you throughout the book.

Unfortunately, MS often strikes people between the ages of 20–40. It affects twice as many women as men. Many speculate that the actual number of people with the disease is much higher than the estimated 400,000, because the disease often goes undiagnosed. One reason for this is denial.

Accepting the Unacceptable

Often people intuitively know when something is seriously wrong with them, but they deny their symptoms and hope and pray that they'll go away. I know I did.

Admitting that you're having unusual symptoms and telling your doctor about your situation is in itself a gutsy step. Seeking a diagnosis requires overcoming fear and facing reality—two intimidating tasks. This was certainly the case for Sara, a woman in her early thirties who spent 12 years fearing that she might have MS. She recalls:

> My college roommate was a nursing student. When I told her about my weird symptoms she said it sounded like MS. We both studied the disease and what I read scared me. Once we suspected MS, fear festered inside me like a wound. For years, when strange symptoms mysteriously appeared, panic would sear through me. Anxiety kept me from going to the doctor. After I was married, my husband finally insisted that I find out why I was so tired and forgetful, and why I sometimes felt numb. It was what I had feared all along—MS.

Sara's story is not unusual. Anxiety makes it tempting to ignore the dizziness, numbness, and other less obvious symptoms of MS. Since many early symptoms are vague and transient, it is easy to be seduced into rationalizing their existence. Marsha, an MS patient in her twenties, explains, "As long as I didn't have a diagnosis, I could pretend I didn't have a problem. It was safer to think it was all in my head, than to face it straight on."

It's not uncommon for us to ignore our instincts and deny that something is wrong with our bodies. However, facing reality is necessary in order to start managing our health. In *Kitchen Table Wisdom,* Dr. Rachel Naomi Remen writes, "In denying our own suffering, we may never know our strength or our greatness." We must listen to what our bodies are telling us if we're to take care of ourselves. Ultimately, the genesis of our strength and greatness comes through this knowledge.

As scary as it may be to confirm the diagnosis of MS, many feel a deep sense of relief when they finally discover the cause of their mysterious symptoms. Emma, a 38-year-old MS patient, says, "I knew something was wrong. This may sound strange, but getting the diagnosis gave me solace. MS put a name to what I was experiencing and it helped me take a course of action." Clients often instinctively know that they're ill and once someone else verifies it, the flood gates of worry are released and reason can finally take over.

This feeling of relief isn't surprising since living with ambiguity generally causes greater stress than dealing with the facts. An official diagnosis allows people to shift their focus from anxiety and fear toward a proactive treatment plan.

Getting a Diagnosis

As many of you know, even after you've made the decision to explore the cause of your symptoms, it can still be a battle to obtain an accurate diagnosis. Almost every MS patient experiences obstacles while going through the diagnostic process.

In part, this is because most general practitioners find the indicators of MS to be confusing or misleading. Since MS patients report a wide range of symptoms, including memory loss, strange pains, ringing in the ears, difficulty swallowing, clumsiness, confusion, depression, numbness, dizziness, bowel and bladder issues, and vision and balance disturbances, it is easy to understand that these problems can be attributed to many different causes. These ambiguous symptoms often lead to a series of time-consuming tests and inaccurate diagnostic conclusions. As a result, patients frequently leave their doctor's office with more questions than answers, once they have begun their quest to determine the source of their symptoms.

Trust Your Intuition

Shockingly, many of my clients have been told that their problems are psychological rather than physical in nature. In fact, not long ago, many MS patients were actually misdiagnosed as having hysteria. This can be a humiliating and discouraging experience, but you must stay the course and pursue the truth. One determined patient, Nancy, who has lived with MS for five years, describes her ordeal:

> When I first went to my general practitioner to tell him about the numbness in my face, he suggested it was a reaction to stress in my new job. The same doctor told me that the numbness in my legs was caused by wearing ski boots and my dizziness stemmed from an inner-ear infection. He basically implied that it was all in my head. Finally, I went to a neurologist, who immediately suspected MS. After further testing, he confirmed the diagnosis. The worst part of the whole ordeal was that I was beginning to think I was going crazy.

By following her own intuition, Nancy found the truth she was seeking. Even today, some doctors are still hesitant to give the diagnosis of MS. One physician I spoke with was direct and honest about his dread of telling patients they had the disease: "It is difficult to tell someone in the prime of their life that they have a chronic and progressive neurological condition. I tend to take the 'wait and see' approach before sending them on to a specialist." To be fair, until recently it *was* difficult to definitively determine a diagnosis of MS and there were no viable treatment options available. This may have led physicians, as well as patients, to be less vigilant about exploring the possibility that MS could be lurking. Dr. Louis Rosner, author of *Multiple Sclerosis*, writes, "Even when MS has been strongly suspected, many doctors are reluctant to inform the patient of an unconfirmed hunch. Instead, they have been more likely to wait for more signs and symptoms to appear, a process often taking many years."

Fortunately, significant breakthroughs in MS medical research are changing the diagnostic process for the better. Great strides have been made in the last 10 years. Sophisticated magnetic resonance imaging (MRI) techniques are now used in conjunction with spinal taps, clinical histories, and physical exams to more accurately diagnose MS.

Find the Right Doctor

Whether you know you have MS (or you suspect you have the disease and are in the process of seeking a diagnosis), it is critical to find a neurologist who has experience treating MS. Because this is such an unusual disease, it requires specialized training to treat it properly. You should be able to turn to your physician for information, guidance in treatment options, direction in symptom management, and decisions about hospitalization. In addition, your doctor should be able to refer you to other specialists, such as physical therapists, counselors, occupational therapists, and home-health service workers. We will discuss the benefits of many of these services in later chapters.

Most people have to search extensively to find a physician that's right for them, but it is worth the effort. Once you make the right connection, this partnership can play a significant role in reducing your anxiety and supporting your overall sense of well-being.

Personally, I went through four neurologists before I found Dr. Stanley Cohan. He became my trusted adviser and confidant. When my symptoms flared or I had an attack, I knew I could rely on Dr. Cohan's recommendations. Over time, we built a relationship based upon honest communication. This foundation allowed me to rely on him when my judgment was impaired by fear, stubbornness, or cognitive problems. Dr. Cohan acknowledged my symptoms and validated my reactions to those symptoms. His understanding, combined with his expertise in the field of MS, reassured me when the disease had me rattled. Most importantly, I truly felt he cared about me.

As I mentioned in the introduction, the neurologist who initially diagnosed me didn't have the sensitivities and empathy of Dr. Cohan, and his approach caused me a great deal of needless trauma. If you're not currently getting what you need from your doctor, I urge you to find another physician who meets your needs. You deserve to be treated well and to be understood.

To find a qualified doctor, call the National Multiple Sclerosis Society (see the Resources section for contact information) and ask for the names of neurologists in your area who specialize in treating MS. You might also check with your internist, the neurologist who diagnosed you (if they are not an expert in the diagnosis and treatment of MS), local medical schools, and other people you know with MS. I suggest that you meet with a few different physicians to determine if they're a good match. You want to feel that your doctor is approachable and that your questions and concerns are addressed to your satisfaction. At the very least, your new doctor should be current on treatment options, as well as on research in the field of MS. Your choice of neurologist may be the most crucial decision you make in influencing the course of your disease, so take the time to thoroughly research their doctor's credentials.

Get to Know Your Symptoms

Obtaining an accurate diagnosis will be dependent on the physician's skill and experience, but it will also be dependent on your ability to explain the changes you have noticed in your body. Whether you are still searching for a definitive diagnosis, or whether you're currently trying to better manage your disease, you will want to mention and explain in detail every symptom you've experienced. For instance, when did the symptom start? How long did it last? Did you regain full functioning once the symptom disappeared, or did you experience residual effects? Were your feelings constant or did they fluctuate? Did anything bring you relief?

It is helpful to keep a journal and jot down all these specifics. For example, since heat sensitivity is one of the indicators of MS, tell the doctor if exercising or taking warm baths aggravates your symptoms. Tracking your symptoms will enhance your communication with your doctor and remind you of important details that you tend to forget as you start to feel better.

Some of the more common symptoms of MS include the following:

❖ Increase in reflexes, such as a hyperresponse to a tap on your funny bone

❖ Fatigue that stops you in your tracks

❖ Ataxia (loss of muscle control)

❖ Spasticity (a sensation of tightening or twitching in muscles)

❖ Sensory loss or numbness

❖ Double or blurred vision

❖ Bladder problems, such as frequency or urgency

❖ Dizziness

❖ Speech and swallowing difficulties

❖ Weakness in limbs (feeling as if you have worked a muscle to exhaustion when you're simply trying to push on the gas pedal)

Although the individual presence of any one of these symptoms may not mean you have MS, these are indicators that should be brought to your doctor's attention before or after you've been diagnosed. If you're alarmed by the number of symptoms on this list, take heart in knowing that most people with MS will only experience a few of these problems throughout their lives. Later in the book, you will be given an exercise to help you identify how your symptoms may be influenced by stress, and ways to minimize stress's impact.

In addition to tracking your symptoms and jotting them down, it can be helpful to bring a family member or trusted friend along with you during your medical appointment so that they can contribute to your clinical history. We tend to compensate for our losses. In fact, we can become so skilled at adjusting to our symptoms that we fail to objectively see changes in our abilities. Compensation is a great coping technique, but it can obscure the picture for your doctor. I've been amazed by the observations my husband makes during our visits to the neurologist. He recently said that my limp was more pronounced and I had become forgetful. I wish I'd left him at home that day!

Treatment Is Now Available

The most important reason for getting a definitive diagnosis is that for the first time in history, new medications such as Avonex, Betaseron, Copaxone, Rebif, and Tysabri are available to help slow the progression of the disease and reduce the number of attacks for many MS patients. Although none of these treatments provide a cure, often the sooner you can start on one of these drug therapies, the better your chances are of managing your symptoms and reducing your risk of disability. These new drugs are a tremendous incentive for patients to see their doctor early and explore treatment options. You can't afford to waste precious time when something could be done to change the course of your disease for the better.

If lack of insurance or finances is an obstacle to treatment, explore financial assistance options with these drug companies. Often these manufactures have programs to help make the drugs more affordable. Your neurologist may also know of assistance programs that are available through the drug companies and may be able to help you with the application process.

Easing the Stress of Injections

All of the current disease-modifying medications must be injected. For some, this can also be a stumbling block to treatment. Sticking yourself with a needle is naturally counterintuitive. Most agree, however, that the benefits of the treatments and the knowledge that the patient is doing all they can to battle their illness outweigh the discomfort of the injections. So what can be done to make the task easier?

If you are especially anxious about injections, create a ritual around the procedure. Designate a place in your home where you always take your shot. Be sure the area is warm and well lit. You may want to be in a room where you can lock the door so that no one can barge in and surprise you just as you have gotten up the nerve to go for it. Evenings are often the best time to inject because then you can sleep through the worst of the unpleasant side effects. However, some people are too tired at night and prefer to do it earlier in the day. Choose a time that works best for you and stick with it. (No pun intended.)

Listening to soothing music, lighting candles, and taking a few deep, calming breaths can help you unwind. Some people benefit from a short form of guided imagery to relax the area they are about to inject. For example, you might say, "I see my muscle relaxing ... I feel my warm breath going into the muscle ... I feel calm and confident, and I'm grateful to have this healing treatment enter my body." Our thoughts are what make us anxious, so it stands to reason that they can just as easily be used to help us relax.

The more confident we become about giving ourselves injections, the less nervous we will be. If you have any doubts about your technique, consult with your doctor's office and review the procedure.

One of the best tips I've learned is to use the smallest needle necessary. The current standard needle in the Avonex package is long enough to go through any amount of fat to reach the muscle. I don't have much fat, so I'm able to get away with a 25-gauge, 1-inch needle. The pharmacy will sell you a box of 100, and you simply exchange the larger needle with the smaller one when you are prepping. Check with your doctor to see if using a smaller needle is appropriate in your situation.

Taking acetaminophen or ibuprofen a few hours before you take your shot can reduce both the pain and flu-like side effects that you may experience. If your medication is refrigerated, taking it out of the refrigerator a few hours beforehand can reduce the burning sensation. Icing the injection area on your body also lessens the pain.

After 10 years of injecting myself, I finally gave in and asked my husband to relieve me. I wish I had done this sooner. When he injects me in the arm every few weeks, it gives my thighs (the usual injection site) a welcome reprieve. Those with extreme needle phobias may always prefer to have someone else inject them. I have clients whose neighbors, spouses, and even teenage children learn to administer shots.

Finally, be sure to reward yourself for doing what you can to treat your disease. On shot days, have your spouse make dinner for you, or relax and watch a video. You've earned it.

Combination therapies are also available for those who continue to have break-through episodes or frequent flare-ups despite ongoing treatment. Intravenous steroids can be administered to minimize the effects of an attack. Of course, all these medications have side effects, so the risks versus rewards need to be carefully considered by both you and your doctor.

Unfortunately, some people still believe that nothing can be done for MS. "I didn't go to my doctor for years even though I was pretty sure I had MS," says one woman in her late fifties. "I just couldn't see what the use was in finding out I had something that I couldn't do anything about." Sadly, this misconception causes many people to miss out on the opportunity to benefit from drug therapies earlier in the disease process.

After getting over the initial terror of my diagnosis, I was grateful to realize that with all the medical advances that have occurred recently, there has never been a better time to have MS.

In addition to disease-modifying drugs, there are many medications that can help treat bladder problems, depression, fatigue, insomnia, spasticity and the other symptoms that MS forces us to contend with. These will be discussed in future chapters. With a proper diagnosis and the right doctor, you can begin to make informed decisions about your health care depending on what makes sense for you and your current life situation. Information is power, and power puts you in charge.

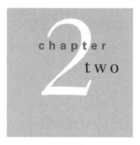

chapter
two

Coming to Terms with MS

I didn't ask for this disease, and now that I have it,
I don't know what to do with it.

— *Kate; age 28, veterinarian, MS patient for 2 years*

Being diagnosed with a chronic illness forces us to confront our own limitations and vulnerabilities. Initially, dealing with MS can feel overwhelming, but eventually you can learn to minimize the impact of the disease and begin to regain a sense of mastery over your life.

One gentleman in his sixties shares his MS experience: "When I was first diagnosed, it was all I thought about. I'd wake up every morning and take an inventory of what was working and what was not. With time, I gained confidence in my body again and without even noticing it, MS started to take more of a backseat in my life. On some level, it is always there, but it no longer takes up all the space in my mind."

Most of us go through a period of getting to know our bodies in an intense, fresh way when we have a serious illness. Initially, we may become hyperaware of every nuance and change that occurs within us—and supersensitive to the symptoms we develop. With time, most people adjust to their "new normal," as they learn how to more accurately read their symptoms and discern what's a serious flare-up and what's just a transient bother. We develop a new rhythm within our bodies that accommodates MS.

Reactions Differ

Although we all respond in our own unique way to hearing that we have MS, there are generally a few typical reactions to the diagnosis. Many go into a "shutdown" mode to deal with the news. Says one newly diagnosed woman, "When I first found out I had MS, I didn't think I could handle it. When I was a kid, I knew one person with MS and she was in a wheelchair so that was what I pictured for myself. I was a 32-year-old woman with two kids. I fell apart. My husband was great, though. He read some of the books that were available and kind of censored them for me, reading the helpful parts out loud and leaving out the scary stuff. I could only take MS in small bites."

Shock is another typical response. Margaret Blackstone, MS patient and author of the book *The First Year of Multiple Sclerosis* points out, "You are right to be shocked by your diagnosis. Shock is a human response that allows the mind to accept the unacceptable gradually, from a psychological distance, rather than being overwhelmed." Shock is a self-protective mechanism that kicks in when we require it. After we're first diagnosed, our belief systems are challenged and our trust in all we once knew is broken. Shock gives us an opportunity to catch up with our reality. Bill, a patient in his mid-forties describes his experience with shock, "When I was first diagnosed, I had this strange physical response during the appointment. I felt as if I went down into a tunnel and my vision narrowed. My doctor's voice faded and sounded far away, sort of like Charlie Brown's mother in the cartoon. It wasn't so much an out-of-body experience, but I definitely tried to pull back from the reality of what was happening. I couldn't hear another word after he said it was MS."

Don't worry. Eventually the shock wears off and you can begin gathering the information you'll need to deal positively with your diagnosis. Even after the initial shock subsides, you may need to learn about the disease gradually and write down questions or concerns as they come up. This strategy allows you to take in what you can at your own pace and enables you to discuss your concerns with your doctor later, when you are calmer and better prepared.

Not all reactions to the disease are negative. Amazingly, many patients find that getting the diagnosis actually serves as a productive turning point in their lives. One client in her mid-forties, Suzanne, says, "For several years I'd been overweight and felt miserable about myself. When I learned I had MS, I just caught fire. I wanted to do everything I could to get healthy. I went to a nutritionist and started walking. I studied the disease and became an expert on my own health. I went from feeling totally out of control to really having a handle on my life. I don't know if I would have made those changes without MS to motivate me."

In some ways, Suzanne's response makes sense. As social worker Wendy Lustbader writes in *Counting on Kindness*, "Illness compels us to confront the difference between the life we had hoped to live and the life we are actually living. Illness accelerates our ventures into neglected aspects of ourselves." Since MS is rarely fatal, it can truly change our perspective at a time when we are still able to positively change the course of our lives.

An MS diagnosis can force you to begin looking more closely at the life choices you make and can influence important life-planning decisions. "We were about to start a family before I got diagnosed," says Jenny, an MS patient in her thirties. "Once we learned I had MS, we decided not to have a child. I know this is a very personal decision, but for us, it was the right one. I am really glad I knew I had MS before going ahead and having a baby."

Knowing that you have MS can make you consider your future in new ways. When you have a potentially disabling, unpredictable illness, you tend to re-evaluate your life. You realize with intense certainty that everything you have always taken for granted can disappear in a heartbeat. This realization can be a burden or a gift depending on how you choose to view it.

Initially, it is not unusual for news of the diagnosis to take people to the most frightening extremes their minds can conjure. Even with all my professional training, I had a complete meltdown after learning I had MS. As a medical social worker, I'd seen the devastation MS could cause and I now saw myself as a patient who was vulnerable and who faced an uncertain future. I cried on my husband's shoulder and said that I wouldn't blame him if he left. I shared the news with the rest of my family and closest friends and saw my own fear reflected back in their eyes. I wish I could tell you that I was gallant or brave or wise, but truthfully, I was a basket case. In retrospect, I realize that all of those feelings were genuine and necessary, that I had to fully experience those despairing moments to begin moving toward acceptance of the disease. But at the time, I just hurt like hell.

Regardless of your initial reaction, absorbing the full blow of an MS diagnosis takes a great deal of emotional processing. Illness humbles us and brings with it many negative associations. It can take a while to let MS become a reality in your life. Part of acknowledging the diagnosis involves a shift in your self-image, and this doesn't happen overnight.

In addition to our own conflicted feelings about being ill, those around us may also have a hard time believing the diagnosis, and their disbelief can add to our difficulty in adjusting. Often, the invisible nature of MS makes the disease extremely difficult for everyone to accept. Initially, it is important to be patient and gentle with yourself and your loved ones as you adjust to this new reality.

Rest assured that whatever your initial response is to the disease, it is likely to be a temporary one. Eventually, you will begin to reshape your identity and establish a new sense of yourself as someone who has MS but who is not consumed by it.

Avoid Impulsive Decisions

Naturally, most people are deeply affected when first diagnosed with a serious chronic condition. Deep thoughts and profound fears will flood your mind initially; however, I caution you to take heed. Restrain yourself from making any major life-altering decisions for at least the first year after you've been diagnosed. You need time to gain perspective and develop an understanding of the implications of your diagnosis. Since the course of MS is so variable, you can't make assumptions about how it will affect you until you've lived with it for a little while—and even then, things can change. Unfortunately, patients may make hasty decisions that they later regret. Some quit their jobs shortly after getting MS, even when they're still perfectly able to work. One of my clients sold a house that she loved in order to buy a more practical one-level ranch. Many years later, she's still walking without so much as a limp and laments her decision. Unless your symptoms force you to make an immediate change, give yourself time to adjust to your new condition.

Your Reaction

You might want to take a moment now to fill out the following questionnaire. This exercise will help you examine your own feelings about being diagnosed. I also encourage your family members to write about how they felt when you got the diagnosis. Sharing your responses to the questionnaire can be an effective way to start discussing how you feel about MS coming into your lives.

This exercise is the first of many recommended in this book. I suggest you use a notebook or loose-leaf binder for this and the other exercises in the book that are marked with **; you will have more space in which to write and can add new information and thoughts later. Most likely, you will get the greatest benefit from the following chapters if you do the exercises in the order suggested. This is also a great time to start keeping a journal.

MS DIAGNOSIS QUESTIONNAIRE **

When you were first diagnosed with MS, how did you feel?

Have your feelings changed since you first heard the news?

What were some of your concerns or fears after initially being diagnosed?

What questions did you have?

Did you want to talk with others about it?

How did others respond to learning that you had MS?

MS DIAGNOSIS QUESTIONNAIRE FOR LOVED ONES

When your loved one was first diagnosed with MS, how did you feel?

Have your feelings changed since you first heard the news?

What were some of your concerns or fears after learning of the diagnosis?

What questions did you have?

Did you want to talk with others about it?

How did others respond to learning that your loved one had MS?

It's Time to Talk

If you take the time to complete this exercise and do it with someone who cares about you, it can be a powerful therapeutic experience. Clients have used this tool as a catalyst to begin meaningful discussions that seemed difficult to start without the structure of the exercise. One woman who had lived with the disease for almost two years says, "I thought I knew how I felt about getting the diagnosis, but once I started writing I was shocked by all the feelings that came out. I had stuffed a lot of my emotions to protect my partner. Instead of protecting her, I was alienating her. When we did the exercise together, we really started talking about how the disease was affecting us, instead of ignoring it. For the first time we both felt that we had to deal with the disease together and this made us stronger as a couple."

In *Climbing Higher,* talk show host Montel Williams, diagnosed with MS in 1999, writes, "I think more marriages would be preserved if people were 100 percent open about the disease from the beginning, rather than taking months to get to the same point, after the damage has already been done. Otherwise your spouse feels left out, like you're closing up and you're pushing them away."

Although getting an MS diagnosis can be a terribly lonely experience, when we allow ourselves to feel the support of others, our burden is lessened and we feel more connected to those we love. Doing this exercise together encourages a feeling of partnership as you both attempt to cope with the ramifications of this disease.

As the old saying goes, "A joy shared is doubled, a sorrow shared is halved."

However, when doing this exercise, be prepared. Your loved one could express feelings or thoughts that surprise or even hurt you initially. You may also discover some powerful reactions of your own that you were unaware of previously. Once you complete the exercise, I suggest that you share your answers one at a time. You may want to go first. This way you will not be interrupted or distracted while doing the exercise. Take some time to absorb what the other is saying.

Talking honestly can be tough work and feel awkward, but pretending that nothing is wrong is unhealthy for everyone. As you become more comfortable talking openly about your disease, you may find it easier to cope with many other aspects of MS.

The Future Looks Promising

In the early stages after the diagnosis, a great deal of anxiety is often caused by preconceived notions about MS. If you know someone who has MS, you might immediately assume that their condition will be the same as yours. Perhaps you've seen stars on television, such as Annette Funicello, struggling with the disease and you envision yourself battling the same symptoms. Confusion and misunderstanding about MS are prevalent because the disease affects everyone differently. Although it is difficult to predict the course of your illness, most doctors agree that the first five to seven years of your disease will be a good predictor of your future prognosis.

As Dr. Cohan mentions in his Foreword, when left untreated, the disease will typically progress. However, we're now seeing that treatment can have a significant impact on the course of the disease. You may be fortunate enough to be part of the new generation of MS patients who benefit from the new disease-modifying drugs that are now available. Because these treatments have been developed so recently, we don't yet have statistics to reflect how these breakthroughs will actually improve long-term outcomes. One can only assume that our odds will be improved.

Of course, statistics are one thing and living intimately with the disease is another. Initially, you can expect the diagnosis to have a significant emotional impact on you regardless of the physical consequences you experience.

Acceptance Is Not Quitting

No matter what your initial reaction is to having MS, your ability to eventually gain a healthy perspective on living with the disease must begin with acceptance. Without acceptance, a tremendous amount of energy can be squandered while you are trying to deny the existence of the disease. No matter how hard we try to deny it, the illness continues to exist and the positive energy that could be directed toward managing MS is diluted. Wasted energy is simply a luxury that few people with MS can afford.

Frequently, the notion of acceptance is confused with surrender or giving in, but in fact, acceptance is what allows you to regain a sense of control over your life and your disease. The definition of acceptance is "to regard as true and to take upon oneself the duties and responsibilities of." By fully accepting the diagnosis of MS, you begin to take responsibility for your health. It becomes your duty to learn all you can about the disease and how to manage it. Acceptance gives you the opportunity to begin making the best of what life has to offer you. It's not an excuse to throw up your hands and quit.

As you might expect, acceptance is a goal to work toward, not a state of grace that comes automatically. Our degree of acceptance will fluctuate just like our symptoms fluctuate. However, the fact that you're reading this book indicates that you've reached a certain level of acceptance. How will you know when you've truly come to terms with having MS? In my own experience, this occurred when I stopped expecting myself to be exactly as I was and started cutting myself some slack, making allowances for the changes that had occurred in my abilities. Acceptance means something different for each of us. Dr. Rosner, author of the book *Multiple Sclerosis*, offers a ten-point checklist that outlines some of the indicators of disease acceptance. I've adapted this list in the hope that you might view these steps as positive goals to work toward.

DISEASE ACCEPTANCE

MS is no longer the focus of your life.

Sadness, anger, and disappointment are occasional emotions, not a way of life.

Although you're optimistic, you accept that the disease may progress in the future.

You continue to make plans for the future based on your current level of ability, with the understanding that these plans may need to be altered.

In the event of physical impairment, you're able to readjust your goals in work, play, and relationships to match your ability.

You're no longer consumed by fear of the future.

You're willing to accept help from others, while finding your own way to reciprocate.

Regardless of physical limitations, you strive to maintain a positive self-image.

You follow good health practices and avoid tempting fate with factors that can aggravate your condition.

You view MS as an added challenge in your life, and not merely as the reason for all your problems.

Achieving these goals is a tall order, but having specific targets to shoot for can be inspiring. Many techniques suggested in this book are designed to help you gain a healthier acceptance of your disease.

Living with Uncertainty

After being diagnosed, most patients wonder, "What will having MS mean for me?" Unfortunately, because this question can't be answered definitively, many feel frustrated and fearful. Wondering "What if . . . ?" can cause a tremendous amount of needless anxiety for patients—because at this point, we are unable to accurately predict the course of the disease and what may come. It can be helpful to remind yourself that you've learned to live with uncertainty in other areas of your life, and you can also learn to tolerate the unpredictability of MS.

You can alleviate some of the anxiety by focusing on what you *do* have control over. None of us have any guarantees in life, but we do get to choose how we approach our lives, day to day. Making the decision to deal with your MS proactively and positively is your best assurance that tomorrow will be a better day. The following Sanskrit prayer brings this point home: "Yesterday is but a dream, tomorrow is only a vision. But today, well lived, makes every day a dream of happiness and every tomorrow a vision of hope."

Feeling Numb?

Awakening Your Inner Life

After a while, I became afraid to have any feelings. I was
worried that strong emotions, good or bad, would bring
on symptoms. I just began to hold it all in.

— Niki; 29-year-old housewife, mother of two,
MS patient for three years

Stuffing It

Most of us are clear about the connection between taking care of
our bodies and feeling healthier. We try to exercise and watch our
diets. We drag ourselves to the doctor when we have symptoms.
We take medications or use alternative therapies. In general, we're
willing to do whatever it takes to improve our condition. But when
it comes to taking care of our emotional health, we are often ne-
glectful. For many of us, our feelings become like annoying children—we tend to ignore them and hope they'll go away. However,
when we fail to honor our internal messages, we miss a powerful
opportunity to enhance our physical well-being and manage our
symptoms better.

In recent years, a strong correlation has been discovered between our emotions and our health. Dr. Candace Pert, respected scientist and author of *Molecules of Emotion*, writes about the importance of attending to our feelings: "The tendency to ignore our emotions is *oldthink*, a remnant of the still-reigning paradigm that keeps us focused on the material level of health, the physicality of it. But the emotions are a key element in self-care because they allow us to enter into the bodymind's conversation. By getting in touch with our emotions, both by listening to them and by directing them through (our body), we gain access to the healing wisdom that is everyone's natural biological right."

As Dr. Pert's research indicates, we're equipped with emotions for a reason. Feelings guide us toward health and wholeness, so when we neglect our emotional life, we become lost. This was the case for Niki, an attractive woman in her thirties. Niki's hair was cut into a smart bob, her makeup was expertly applied, and her clothes elegantly draped over her well-toned frame. Externally, she presented the image of a sophisticated and urbane professional woman who had things under control. But I sensed that something was amiss. Niki seemed frozen. Her smile was tight and her laugh was nervous. In her effort to maintain control, she was losing it. Her outsides didn't match her insides.

Initially, we had trouble connecting. "Tell me what brought you here today? What would you like to discuss?" I asked. And she began, "I guess the issue is that I have MS. I was diagnosed two years ago. I'm doing okay physically, but I get really tired so I cut back my hours at work. I have some bladder problems and numbness and optic neuritis issues, but I'm really doing well." Niki went on in great detail about how MS had started to limit her activities. She also mentioned that it was impacting her relationship with her husband; however, she would always end her sentences with a quick, insincere smile, saying, "but I really can't complain; I'm doing very well."

Steering away from discussing her physical symptoms, I began to explore how she was feeling emotionally. "What do you mean how am I emotionally?" she asked. I said, "Well, you've described to me a life that has changed dramatically. Your income has been reduced, your marriage is strained, you're no longer able to play sports with your friends, and you're constantly up at night going to the bathroom; so, how do you feel about all this?" "It could be a lot worse," she replied.

This answer sums up how Niki was dealing with her disease. Every time she told herself that her condition could be worse, she cut off her ability to experience any natural feelings of anger, sadness, or frustration. She edited out her emotional life. Although not all patients respond this way, withdrawing emotionally is a common coping technique among MS patients. In Niki's case, she reasoned that since her MS could be worse, she had no right to complain or have feelings about how difficult it was now. Along with all the other physical losses Niki was experiencing, she had also lost her ability to feel legitimate grief. At first glance, this emotional distancing appeared to reflect a positive attitude, but in reality, it made Niki feel like a hollow shell of her true self.

Eventually, with tears in her sad blue eyes, Niki admitted that she thought she was getting off easy because her symptoms hadn't put her into a wheelchair. She actually felt guilty for not being more disabled than she was: "I feel like if I complain or give in to how I feel, I might get worse. I don't want to throw myself a pity-party." The determination not to complain because others have it worse is another way that MS patients switch off their emotions. Of course, someone will *always* have it better or worse than you, but that doesn't mean that your experience isn't meaningful or valid.

Don't get me wrong. Naturally, there are times when we benefit from comparing our situations with others. Comparisons can allow us to put our situation into perspective. But when we use comparisons to minimize our own difficult feelings, we inhibit our ability to move through and beyond our pain. We have no chance of getting to the other side of an emotion if we don't allow ourselves to recognize and express our experience. Keeping our concerns to ourselves can lead to destructive feelings that can become suppressed and turned inward.

There is also social pressure to suffer in silence. In *Brandished Knowledge* Alice Miller explains, "Not to take one's own suffering seriously, to make light of it, or even laugh at it, is considered good manners in our culture. This attitude is even called a 'virtue.'" Unfortunately, society reinforces a stoic stance. We're taught that it is better to keep our "complaints" to ourselves. But the price we pay is isolation. Keeping up a good front inevitably makes us feel distant and misunderstood by others, rather than accepted and loved, as we so desire.

MS limits us enough physically, so it shouldn't cripple us emotionally as well.

Looks Can Be Deceiving

Niki also did a good job of convincing others that she was fine. Based on appearance, she looked like the picture of health. But looks can be deceiving. A frequent frustration among MS patients is to be told, "But you look so good," after revealing that they have MS or mentioning that they're experiencing symptoms. This response, although well intended, devalues our pain and can make us feel ashamed or discounted by others. Niki explains, "It's as if people expect you to look awful or use a cane or a wheelchair, and if you don't, then your symptoms aren't really serious." Once you get the "But you look so good" response a few times, you begin to feel that you should keep silent about your symptoms, unless you look like a train wreck. This can be a deeply demoralizing experience.

Although most of us will experience a serious disease at some point in our lives, many people generally still don't know how to respond kindly to the illness of another. When they can't find words of comfort, they may insensitively say the first thing that comes to mind. To add insult to injury, the uncomfortable reactions of friends and family to your disease can make it more difficult for you to accept your own feelings about being sick. Keep in mind that although they may struggle to comprehend your illness, many people are simply unable to respond with genuine solace. Their apparent lack of empathy or understanding says more about *their own* inability to reach out than it does about your illness.

Niki's experience illustrates this point. Because Niki looked so well and tried to maintain the role of the "good patient" who never complained, she lost touch with how she actually felt about being ill. To help Niki regain a connection with her inner voice, I asked her to speak one word to describe how she felt about having MS. She was slow to respond, and her face turned crimson as she pushed back her hair and sputtered, "Cheated." Of course, Niki had to add, "But others have it much worse." I stopped her. I said, "I want you to tell me that you feel cheated and stop there, with no disclaimers." Eventually, Niki was able to say how she felt without sugarcoating it.

This was a good start. It was the beginning of Niki's acknowledgement of how she actually felt—of her sense that MS was robbing her of part of her life. She had to recognize and admit her pain before she could reclaim her emotional self, if not her physical self, from the disease. As long as there was no problem, there was no solution.

Take a moment now to choose *one* word that describes how you feel about having MS, and enter it on the following line:

_____

Feelings Never Vanish; They Only Hibernate

On further reflection, Niki realized that she had not always been so disconnected from her emotional life: "I think what I've learned is that since my diagnosis, anytime I get upset or even excited about positive things like when we bought our new house, my symptoms go haywire. I try to keep myself calm because if I get nervous or angry I can feel my face or legs start to go numb. I just can't afford to have anything else go wrong. I have become so attuned to these triggers that after a while I've trained myself not to 'go there' because it means that I would pay the price with more symptoms."

It is common for MS patients to gradually start ignoring their feelings in a misguided attempt to manage their symptoms. Like Niki, they associate intense emotions with exacerbations. Just as you learn to avoid a hot stove to keep from getting burned, you may also learn to ward off conflict, sadness, or anger, in an effort to preserve your health. Unfortunately, this can backfire on you.

During her intensive scientific research regarding the body-mind connection, Dr. Pert discovered the following about our emotions: "All honest emotions are positive emotions. All emotions are healthy because emotions are what unite the mind and body. Anger, fear, sadness, the so-called negative emotions are as healthy as peace, courage, and joy. To repress these emotions and not let them flow freely is to set up a disintegrity in the system, causing it to act at cross-purposes rather than as a unified whole. The stress this creates is what sets up the weakened condition that can lead to disease." In summary, it is the effort we exert in holding back our emotions that actually makes us more susceptible to disease. We suffer significant consequences by ignoring our emotions.

Pam, a 36-year-old mother of three, felt deeply conflicted about expressing her feelings: "When going through my divorce, I was furious that my husband was leaving me. I felt abandoned, frightened, and outraged that after all we had gone through he could be so heartless. But every time we would start to argue, my vision would get blurry and my head would start to buzz. I just knew it would make me sick to keep fighting. I felt like I couldn't risk getting upset so I became pitifully apathetic. He ended up taking advantage of me in the worst way."

Our task is not to avoid feelings, but to learn how to manage them. It wasn't until she came into therapy that Pam was able to honestly express her emotions. By developing conscious techniques to thoughtfully express her feelings, she minimized the effects her anger and frustration had on her symptoms.

The first step Pam took was to recognize that she was avoiding her feelings because she had literally become afraid of them. Pam learned that by writing down her concerns either in a diary or in letters to her ex-husband, she was able to avoid getting swept up in the moment and overwhelmed by the immediate conflict. Discussing things earlier in the day also helped her to stay focused and become less upset. "It seemed like we would always try to discuss things at night when I was exhausted and not thinking clearly. After 7:00 P.M., I didn't have the energy to have an intelligent conversation, much less a debate with my husband," she observed. Pam also found that using a recorder when she and her husband had difficult conversations allowed her to feel more confident. These small changes allowed Pam to experience her feelings without being at their mercy.

It is ironic that when we attempt to avoid experiencing our emotions in order to protect our health, we may actually exacerbate physical problems. In fact, experts now say that from 60 to 90 percent of all doctor visits involve stress-related complaints. The root of most stress comes from repressed emotions that leave us feeling conflicted.

Consider Clark, a 62-year-old business owner who came to me with complaints of headaches, insomnia, anxiety, and nausea. Walking into my office with the help of a cane, Clark appeared to be a dignified and composed gentleman. He stated, "I've lived with MS for about 10 years. It has slowed me down a bit, so I've passed my business on to my son. Now I play a little golf. My wife is still working, so I try to make myself useful around the house. She gets upset if she thinks I overdo it, so I guess life has become a bit dull." I asked Clark when he started to get the headaches and have trouble sleeping; he said it happened about two years ago. His symptoms began when he turned his business over to his son. As it turned out, Clark was not ready to retire, but his wife and son pushed for it because they didn't want him to become further disabled by the MS. They had decided to retire Clark and he went along with it because he didn't want to "rock the boat." "What if I did keep working and ended up getting sicker? It wouldn't be fair to my family," he explained.

With further exploration, Clark revealed that he felt guilty about being slowed down by his disease, but he thought that he was still able to contribute and be effective in his job. It wasn't until he quit working that he began to feel useless. Now his guilt was compounded by anger toward his family for pushing him in this direction, even though they intended for the change to be in his best interest. "How can I be angry at them? They were only trying to do what is best for me," he remarked. But Clark *was* angry. He was angry at having the disease, and he was angry that everyone else continued to go about their lives, leaving him alone to putter around the house. He was angry that he hadn't voiced his feelings. He was literally making himself sick with stifled emotions.

Clark admitted that when he had tried to discuss his feelings with his wife in the past, they would both become very emotional, "and that isn't good for me," he added. Clark noted that his legs would become weak when he got frustrated or angry, "Better just to let these things go and stay even-keeled." This became his mantra. But the words he told himself weren't matching up with his feelings. He wasn't ready to let go. He didn't feel even-keeled and he needed to find a way to express this without bringing on symptoms.

Getting all of his feelings out on the table in our session was a good start for Clark. He realized that his ego had been hurt. He sensed that his family no longer valued him. In addition to missing his work, he no longer felt productive. He also recognized that his guilt over having MS had made him feel as if he had no right to speak up for what he wanted. "I have been holding in more than I thought—for longer than I thought," he remarked with surprise.

It took a while for Clark to get to the core of his issues and recognize that just because he had MS, he didn't have to become a passive bystander in his own life. Naming his feelings and discussing his experience enabled him to identify a variety of emotions—sadness, regret, and hope—that he had been feeling, and as a result, his anger seemed less threatening.

Clark took a further positive step by discussing these issues with his wife, revealing that he was avoiding conflict because he was afraid that it would harm his health. This helped her to respond to him in a more understanding and loving way. The door opened, inviting in better communication. Fewer emotions were bottled up. In addition, Clark was able to improve communication with his son and they agreed that he would act as a consultant at the company. Not surprisingly, as Clark became less conflicted about his feelings and began to express himself, his physical complaints improved.

Psychological Numbness

Symptoms can also rise when life gets interesting. Clients report experiencing exacerbations during both good and bad times (any situation that involves an intense emotion or response); negotiating for a raise, getting cut off by another driver, giving a presentation, scolding the children, buying a new home, taking a long-anticipated vacation, going to a doctor's appointment, grieving the death of a loved one, or getting married. Susie remembers, "I'd been looking forward to my tenth high school reunion for months. Every day my girlfriends and I would chat on the phone about who would be there. I was so looking forward to this party. My hair was cut and colored, I spent a fortune on a great outfit, I lost weight, all the arrangements were made, and then wham, I was knocked broadside by an attack of vertigo. I'm pretty certain that my excitement brought on these symptoms. Now I'm afraid to look forward to anything."

It is heartbreaking to see how the fear of exacerbations causes some MS patients to withdraw from life in an attempt to avoid being vulnerable. If we stop engaging in life and keep our feelings in check, we lose touch with our inner self, which ironically is the psychological equivalent of going numb.

When you have MS, any intense experience may trigger an attack, but climbing into a shell and hiding from life won't insulate you from illness. The roller coaster of life cannot be avoided. Once you're born, you're strapped in and along for the ride, so you might as well throw your arms up in the air and experience the rush. Feelings are to be felt. Life is to be lived. It is messy, it's fun, it's painful, it's extraordinary, it's everything in-between, but it's not to be missed because you're fearful of having a relapse. Rather than hiding from feelings, the successful strategy is to become more aware of them. This awareness allows you to manage emotions and situations in a proactive manner.

Take a moment to determine if you experience a relationship between your emotions and your MS flare-ups. Think about events that may have preceded a previous MS attack. I encourage you to keep a journal and make notes periodically, especially when you have a flare-up. Write down what was going on in your life at the time of your last exacerbation. The following is an example:

Preceding Event: Week-long visit with in-laws; several conflicts and arguments.

Nature of Symptoms: Extreme fatigue requiring bed rest for two days; optic neuritis.

Duration of Symptoms: Fatigue lasted for several days; optic neuritis lasted two months.

If you've recognized a connection between your feelings and your symptoms, ask yourself how you've responded to this. Do you try to avoid conflicts? Do you hold your emotions in? Do you try to make things easier by just sucking it up when you feel blue or frustrated or furious or sick?

As part of your MS symptom management plan, I suggest that you keep an ongoing record of the *feelings* that you have preceding an attack. If you can remember, write about what was going on for you emotionally *prior* to the symptoms, and what emotions came on *during* and *after* the attack. Writing these feelings down may help you diffuse their intensity without avoiding them all together. You should also begin to recognize emotional patterns or triggers that make you more vulnerable to possible exacerbations, and this will help you gain a sense of control over these triggers.

What Do Feelings Feel Like?

If this is the first time you've asked yourself these questions, then like Niki, it may be difficult to determine how you actually experience your feelings. Have you ever seen the chart in your doctor's office, "How Are You Feeling Today?" with all the different circles of faces wearing different expressions? These charts help simplify the process of identifying emotions. If we were all clear on how we felt all the time, the doctor wouldn't need such a chart.

To illustrate how we process our feelings, Dr. Nathaniel Branden, author of *Six Pillars of Self-Esteem,* describes the way we take in our emotions:

> The act of experiencing and accepting our emotions is implemented through (1) focusing on the feeling or emotion, (2) breathing gently and deeply; allowing muscles to relax, allowing the feeling to be felt, and (3) [becoming conscious and therefore] making real the awareness that this is *my* feeling.
>
> In contrast, we deny or disown our emotions when we (1) avoid awareness of their reality, (2) constrict our breathing and tighten our muscles to cut off or numb feeling, and (3) disassociate ourselves from our own experience.

The next time an emotion comes up for you, try to notice how you react to it, not only intellectually, but physically as well. If you're avoiding intense feelings, you may want to work toward changing that pattern. When we resist our reality, we fail to find relief.

As you begin to identify your feelings, you may notice that they serve many purposes. Emotions can be an important guide in showing us what we need to do differently in our lives. "Once I realized how resentful I was about taking on all the chores in our house, I was able to work with my husband to create a plan and solve the problem. He was happy to split up some of the work and hire some help. This simple step probably saved us from getting divorced down the road, and I am sure it's improved my health," recalls one MS patient.

When we view feelings as protective messengers, they take on a whole new meaning. My experience with clients has shown that it is only after they begin to acknowledge their emotions, rather than play them down, that they begin to live well with their disease.

Emotions don't only serve as internal guides; they actually play a vital role in our survival. They generate actions that satisfy needs and protect us from threat and loss. In fact, emotions are often the driving force behind positive actions. We need our emotions to motivate us. Put simply, when we fail to embrace our emotions, we miss an opportunity to take care of ourselves.

Paying attention to emotions also enables you to view your physical symptoms as a source of strength instead of a sign of weakness. That tingling in your legs can be a cue that you need to go inside yourself and assess what you're experiencing and why. Perhaps you need to remove yourself from a stressful situation, take a nap, or reduce your exercise for that day. You can use your MS symptoms as a tool to become more conscious of your feelings and how they are affecting your body. This provides an opportunity to become more insightful and more deliberate in your choices, rather than just reacting impulsively to situations as many of us do.

You *Can* Cope

As you become more aware of your feelings, it is important to feel confident in your ability to handle them. Gaining a clear understanding of your unique coping style will build your confidence. Which of the following coping techniques best describes how you cope with problems, a new situation, or strong feelings?

THE REFLECTIVE

Ask yourself; are you the type that's reflective? Perhaps you need time to process information and allow new thoughts and feelings to sink in. You may tend to spend time alone, reading or researching. Too much external stimulation may overwhelm you. Do you have a high need to control your environment? Do you prefer to react slowly when confronted with a problem or a new situation? If so, then honor your way of dealing with things and ask that others respect your need to mull things over. Don't be pressured into feeling like you must react right away when emotions come up. Give yourself permission to take a time-out when a conversation becomes too heated. In other words, use your natural reflective instincts to get you through tough emotional times.

THE ASSERTIVE

On the other hand, your style may be more assertive. Are you happiest when you are decisive and take action? Do you deal with a problem head-on, possibly trying several different solutions at once? Perhaps your anxiety is eased only when you're actively working to remedy a situation. For you, it may feel better to address an emotional concern right away. If this is your style, you experience a sense of relief once you've set out a course of action and begin to follow it. For instance, if you are feeling anxious about a medical issue, you may want to meet with your doctor right away. Just making the call to schedule an appointment will help you feel better.

THE CONNECTOR

Many people gain solace from sharing with others and interacting socially. Folks with this coping style tend to gravitate toward support groups or a strong network of friends or family to help them face a crisis. If this describes you, you're someone who picks up a phone and calls a friend when you're down in the dumps—and talks through whatever feelings you may be having. You'll want to identify at least three people you know you can call when you need to talk and then tape their names and numbers to the refrigerator for quick and easy access.

See if you can determine what coping style feels right for you. All of us are faced with challenges and difficult feelings during the course of our lives. We've all had to get through hard times in the past, so think back and consider what worked for you then? We all have the capacity to develop internal fortitude and strength to deal with what life throws at us, even if that means relying on others for a while. You just have to become acquainted with your own source of power.

Dr. Linda Miller, a psychologist who treats MS patients, says:

> The essence of coping comes from self-awareness. This can be achieved through relationships with others, writing and journaling, psychotherapy, movement and body therapy, spending time meditating, being in nature, and whatever else

helps people to get to know themselves. I think that increasing self-awareness and self-knowledge is the most important and valuable aspect of accepting and coping with MS. This is an opportunity people without MS often fail to recognize.

Get to Know Yourself

How does living with MS make you feel? Use the following exercise to begin identifying your feelings. If you've lived with the disease for a while, describe how you currently feel about having this condition and how it impacts your life. I recommend doing this exercise at home, at a time when you have no demands placed on you. Like the previous exercise, filling in these answers can stir up many feelings and you need to allow yourself time and space to process your emotions. Again, you may choose to share your answers with a loved one to help them better understand what you're going through. If you feel overwhelmed while answering these or any other questions posed in this book, consider working through your answers with a mental-health professional.

MY MS EXPERIENCE *

How would you describe what it is like to have a chronic illness to someone else?

What have been some of your greatest challenges in facing this disease?

How do you feel about the invisibility of the disease?

What happens when you speak openly with your loved ones about the illness and its impact on you?

How has your life been changed by this disease?

What have you had to give up because of this illness?

What are your greatest fears about the illness?

What have you gained as a result of this disease?

What advice would you give someone who is newly diagnosed?

What impact has this disease had on your relationship with others?

Describe the way you communicate with those close to you about this disease.

What do you think are some common misunderstandings about your illness?

What do you keep from your loved ones, if anything, in order to spare their feelings or protect them?

When do you feel most supported by others in dealing with your illness?

Has your disease affected you positively, and if so, how?

What causes the most misunderstandings about your disease?

What have you felt to be most helpful in coping with your condition?

Is there anything that you haven't expressed to anyone about having this disease? Why have you kept this to yourself?

How has having this illness affected your self-esteem?

What changes have you made in your life to accommodate or adapt to your diagnosis?

What do you want others to know about this disease?

What do you think your spouse or significant other would say about how your illness has affected them?

The answers you provide to these thought-provoking questions will help give a voice to the feelings you have about living with MS. By taking the time to articulate your true feelings about having MS, you start to honestly face how it impacts your entire being. Once you're completely honest with yourself about your relationship with MS, you begin to take power away from the disease and redirect it toward a stronger sense of self. As you better understand the emotions that dwell in your heart, the struggle to hold these feelings in can cease, bringing you much-needed peace and calm.

Clients report that doing this exercise with a loved one brings forth an intense wave of relief and validation. Tim, a thirty-something PR executive remarks:

> My wife, Teresa, finally understood why I'd become so introverted. I was trying to protect her from all the pain and fear I was feeling. I didn't want to make it worse for her, so I just bit my tongue and put up a brave front. Once I started talking to her about my insecurities, and about my concerns about ultimately losing her, she was able to tell me how scared she was for both of us. My aloofness was causing her more agony than if I had just told her how scared I was of what might happen to me, to us. After we talked, she said she hadn't felt that much intimacy with me since I was diagnosed three years ago. We also started to talk realistically about what we'd do if I did become disabled, or if *she* might become disabled. This made us both feel calmer. We started to feel like a team again.

Of course, identifying your feelings and bringing them to the surface can be a demanding endeavor. In the next chapter, we explore ways to make this process easier by teaching you specific skills to augment your coping abilities.

Positive Solutions to Negative Emotions

I never knew I had so many feelings until I got MS.

— Colette; age 39, writer, MS patient for 6 years

Whether you're just now getting in touch with your feelings about MS or whether you've been wearing your heart on your sleeve since day one, MS can create a hell storm of emotions for us all. Patients must deal with the daily fatigue and frustrating unpredictability of the disease, side effects from medications, and the potential physiological effects of demyelination in areas of the brain that regulate mood. The chronic nature of the disease forces us to face a lifetime of challenges (often beginning at a young age). The struggle to continually adjust to physical losses and disabilities can make even the most good-natured person act like Jack Nicholson in *The Shining*. Add steroids to the mix and look out! It is no wonder that many people with MS report battling depression, anger, frustration, impatience, fear, low self-esteem, and periods of grief.

Not surprisingly, it is easy to feel overwhelmed by all the emotions that MS triggers. At times you may be swept away by your reactions to the disease and long for a way to regain control of your emotional life. Libby, a 39-year-old woman with MS who has had the disease for six years, recalls, "I used to be an easygoing, relaxed person, and I rarely lost my temper. Now I'm snapping at everyone. I constantly get frustrated and irritated; then I see how I'm acting and I feel so guilty. But it's too late; the damage is done."

Fortunately, we don't need to be bullied by our own thoughts and feelings. Although there's no formula for coping that's right for everyone, there are some time-tested and effective strategies that may help you take charge of your emotions. As you learn how to manage some of the more difficult psychological reactions to MS, you'll also see improvements in how you manage your disease.

Naming and Sharing Your Feelings

Let's begin with Sharon's story. Sharon is a 45-year-old woman who has been living with MS for nearly twenty years. In the past two years, her condition has worsened. She says, "What I don't understand is why I'm feeling so overwhelmed *now?* I feel angry and irritable and I'm short with my family. I knew that my disease would get worse over time. I've dealt with it for years, but all of the sudden I feel like I can't handle it." I asked Sharon to take a step back and look at everything that was going on in her life, other than the new symptoms that were causing her to use a cane. She replied, "My two girls are in college now. One is about to graduate and the other one will graduate next year. It was our dream to see them get their degrees. One is going on to medical school! But it's been very hard to see them grow up and leave. I've always been able to depend on them. We were, are, very close. I feel empty not having them around."

It soon became apparent that Sharon felt extremely conflicted about her daughters' departure. They were moving ahead with their lives and fulfilling the family's dreams, but Sharon also felt that she was being left behind. As it turns out, her new symptoms brought up feelings of dependency and neediness and deep down she felt abandoned by her girls: "I guess having them at home always gave me a sense of security and a safety net." Once these thoughts and feelings came to the surface, we could begin to deal with them. Sharon decided to explain to her daughters and her husband that she felt lonely and scared by her new symptoms. Her daughters were able to reassure her that they'd be there for her if she ever needed anything. They decided to schedule regular visits and take turns coming home. One daughter told her that she planned to move back to their hometown after graduation. These discussions brought Sharon a great deal of relief.

Next, we looked at ways that Sharon's husband could provide the emotional support that she usually got from her daughters. The couple was able to recognize a pattern that had shut the husband out, as the women in the family rallied around each other. Sharon's husband was eager to meet his wife's needs. It turns out that he was feeling lonely and lost with his daughters being away as well. They helped each other to fill the vacuum caused by their daughters' absence. Now the couple could begin to actually be there for each other.

Sharon's case is a clear example of how letting emotions rise to the surface can start the process of problem solving and healing. Fear of abandonment is a common concern of MS patients. This fear can become a self-fulfilling prophecy if it is not dealt with straight on. Had Sharon not expressed her feelings, she may have continued to act annoyed and irritated with her daughters, pushing them further away. She may have also missed a wonderful opportunity to create intimacy with her husband. Instead, Sharon was able to use her feelings as a way to get more of what she needed. So the first step of managing every difficult feeling is naming it and sharing it.

Taming Fear

Fear was Sharon's underlying emotion, as it is for many MS patients. This is understandable. Few medical conditions paint such an uncertain future, and we're all afraid of the unknown. Living with this disease means living with unpredictability, and when you feel uncertain, it is easy to allow fear to spiral out of control and run your life. But fear doesn't need to enslave you. Fear isn't something to be fixed or ignored. It is to be used as a helpful tool—and then released.

Fear is that rush of adrenaline and pounding in our heart that tells us when we need to act. Our fear can be the motivator that gets us out of a dangerous situation. When we follow our fear to where it leads us, we become empowered to make choices about how we can handle it. Once we take action, fear usually fades and we're released to move on with our lives.

Chronic fear becomes destructive when it leads to a free-floating anxiety that we feel unable to do anything about. When this happens, we need to contain our fear and stop the nonproductive cycle of worrying about things we can't control.

Unfortunately, we never feel more out of control than when our body isn't doing what our mind tells it to do. You may notice that your level of fear will ebb and flow with the severity of your symptoms. In my experience, when you're symptom free, it is easier to reduce fear to a manageable size and to put it on the back burner of your mind. This is much more difficult to do when you're having a flare-up or when you have been recently diagnosed. But this doesn't mean it is impossible.

The next time you're in a state of panic, ask yourself, "Does this fear serve any purpose in my life right now?" In other words, is the fear inviting you to do anything to improve your health—such as getting more sleep or exploring new medication options? Our fear is valuable only when it pushes us to act. If you're simply recycling your feelings of fear and dread and there's nothing positive you can do with the feeling, it is time to reduce fear to a proper size. I'm not suggesting that you can avoid feeling fearful altogether, but as you will see, fear doesn't need to consume you and demand all your attention.

The most frequent fear my clients express is focused on the level of disability they might face in the future. It is normal to wonder what your fate might be, but to continually dwell in that space will paralyze you long before the disease will. There's no way that anyone can predict what the future will be. The best way you can face this issue is to assume that whatever your current level of functioning is today, so it will be tomorrow. If things do change, for better or worse, you can deal with it at the time. An elderly gentleman once gave me some sage advice about living in the moment:

"When you have one foot in yesterday and one foot in tomorrow, you're skipping over today." Wasting quality time fearing what will come next robs you of what joy you might be able to experience in this moment. Before you were diagnosed, did you dwell on all the calamities that might come tomorrow? This type of worry and anxiety doesn't serve you in any way, so let it go.

Fear Is Not Control

Some of us develop a belief that worrying about the future enables us to exert control over what might come. We use fear like a worry stone, turning thoughts over and over, ruminating about what may happen next. Be assured that no matter how much you worry, you won't influence the outcome of future events.

The following sections present some pointers on how to manage fear and worry:

MAKE AN APPOINTMENT WITH FEAR

One way to contain your fear is to set an appointment with it for five minutes each morning and each evening. Actually sit down and commit yourself to worrying from 8:00 A.M. to 8:05 A.M., and then again from 8:00 P.M. to 8:05 P.M. This technique works best if you don't give your fear any more or any less time than the five allotted minutes twice a day. Of course you may still worry at times during the day, but this appointment is the time to intentionally focus on your fears. I have seen surprising success result from this exercise.

One client, Trina, came to see me because she was plagued with worry. Trina's fear of her MS began to consume most of her thoughts. She was tall, thin, and fair skinned, with dark moon-shaped circles under her eyes. While sitting on the couch, she folded her knees up to her chest and wrapped her arms around her long legs. She looked terrified. "I can't stop thinking about all the things that might happen to me with this disease," she cried. "From the minute my eyes open in the morning to the time my head hits the pillow at night, I feel afraid. Sometimes the fear even creeps into my sleep and gives me nightmares." As the old cliché suggests, Trina was "worrying herself sick."

Trina was doubtful when I asked her to make an appointment with her fear, but she made an attempt. After about a month of daily meetings with her anxieties, Trina was stunned: "Not only do I not worry all the time anymore, but I don't even seem to be able to fill the entire five-minute appointments with fears. It seems like all those scary images have just faded away." This is the first exercise I would suggest you try to begin minimizing your own fear.

DILUTE YOUR FEAR

Fear can also be reduced by sharing it with others. When fear is exaggerated or irrational, telling another person about it gives them an opportunity to reassure you and put your concerns into perspective. When I go through a tough time with my symptoms, I forget that eventually I will feel better. I may have a day, a week, or a month when I'm beyond feeling exhausted and need bed rest. Sometimes dizziness invades my equilibrium. This is the symptom I hate most, and when I experience it, I become convinced I will never again feel like my old self. But I do, or at least I improve, or I adjust to my circumstances. Regardless of the outcome, I always adapt and eventually feel less disturbed by my symptoms. Now, when I become afraid that I'll always feel rotten, I ask my husband and friends to remind me that I won't always feel this way. With rest or steroids or simply time, life improves. Their words calm me when I'm unable to calm myself.

MORE TIPS FOR FACING FEAR

It helps to have a short list of what to do when you feel yourself being overcome by destructive fear. This way, you don't have to think about what to do or recall the coping strategies. Try posting these tips on the refrigerator and use at least three of them as soon as you find yourself being carried away by fearful thoughts:

- ❖ Identify why you're feeling afraid. Write your fear down; that is, name it.

❖ Call a friend or loved one and tell them what you're
  feeling.

❖ Ask yourself if you're safe at the moment.

❖ Come back to the facts of your situation—don't let
  assumptions take over.

❖ Avoid negative people or information. Turn off the television or avoid reading the news if these things are
  contributing to your anxiety.

❖ Create a diversion and do an activity that brings you joy.

When you use at least three of these tips, you should feel your
level of anxiety begin to dissipate.

Fear is a universal experience—one that can help us grow if we
learn to respond to it with awareness. Those of us with MS become
experts in accepting the unknown. As we become more practiced
in living with ambiguity, we develop tolerance, and, in turn, we feel
less fear. With experience, we realize that we can face the challenges that are put in front of us, and we develop a quiet assurance
that we will cope with whatever comes our way.

Our greatest weapon against fear of the future is to enjoy the
present for all it is worth.

Lonely Days and Lonely Nights

When you're diagnosed, you realize that this disease is yours alone.
Others may be there to support you, but they're not in your body,
they don't experience your symptoms, and they can only see the
surface of what you endure. These realizations can make you feel
extremely disconnected.

Having MS can cause your illusions of safety and security to
shift. This might be the first serious problem that you've ever had
that you or someone else couldn't solve. Buddhists say that most of
us live in a world of illusion, yet when suffering shatters that illusion, we're forced to come back to ourselves and rediscover our
core. MS gives us the opportunity to do that. It can lead us back to

our authentic selves. While working with clients, I've often seen people discover a greater sense of self after they're confronted with a crisis. Your wholeness exists in you now regardless of your physical health. Integrity and strength come from the realization that there are times in life when you must rely on yourself. By going inward and learning to nurture yourself, you can become your own best companion.

The process of conquering loneliness begins by learning to be there for yourself. This means that you are the one to figure out what you need and that you take responsibility for getting it. If you're feeling alone and isolated, ask, "What do I want? Is it company, sympathy, empathy, a diversion, a good cry?" You're the only one who truly knows what you're craving and how to get it. Until you understand your own needs, no one else will.

MS patients desperately want understanding. When we feel understood, we feel connected. Jennifer, a 42-year-old woman with MS, explains:

> I want someone to really "get" what I'm going through. I want them to understand what it feels like to be so tired I can't brush my teeth. I want my friends to see when I've had enough and that it's time for them to go home. I want them to realize that I can't listen to several people talking at once and to music at the same time, without getting confused. Little kids and all their questions make me irritable; it's just too much. Sometimes I even need for people to speak more softly or slowly. How do I explain this to others without seeming like a jerk?

As I mentioned earlier, much of what occurs to an MS patient is invisible to others, particularly when the problems stem from fatigue, cognitive difficulties, or emotional issues. There's only one way for people to begin understanding what you're going through; you must tell them. Sure, it can be awkward to ask folks to leave after dinner because you're exhausted, but this honesty is far better than faking it and pushing through an evening while feeling irritable and resentful toward your guests. Believe it or not, everyone picks up the tension, even when you think you're successfully hiding your impatience. Some people will understand and appreciate that you have limits, and they will respect that, just as you would respect a diabetic's need to refuse dessert. Some may not. Although this is sad, it can be a gift to know which friends you should invest your time and energy in and which friends you'd be better off without.

When you feel like others just don't get what you're going through, remember that friends and family don't need to directly experience your symptoms for them to feel empathy for you. We're all connected by our struggles, even if they're not the same. We all experience pain, illness, and sadness at some point in our lives. Ultimately, we all want to feel that others care about us. These are universal experiences that are part of being human. Sometimes the best way to get what you need from others is to give it.

Anger Has Its Place

Anger is a recurrent emotion that many MS patients experience. It's understandable—when our desires are thwarted, our bodies fail us, our minds won't function the way they once did, and we're unable to do the work we love, we can become enraged. Add to these frustrations fatigue, pain, vertigo, and the numerous other insults MS can hurl our way, and it is easy to see why we might feel irate.

Furthermore, MS itself can cause mood swings and irritability. As mentioned earlier, your emotional state can be directly affected by the demyelination occurring in your brain. Depending on where the lesions are located, this can lead to emotional outbursts.

So our anger is justified, but how do we make it work *for* us rather than against us? As long as we retain our mental faculties, we can choose the way we respond to anger. Rather than lashing out at our doctors or loved ones, we can develop strategies that help us release anger in more productive ways.

We've already discussed the importance of experiencing our feelings, but managing anger can be a particular challenge. We may find that we don't know how to express anger other than by having an outburst and then suffering undesirable consequences. When we don't clearly voice our complaints or frustrations, we often don't get what we want from others. This can be maddening, increasing our sense of injustice and rage, and we may end up alienating those we'd hoped to draw closer. However, there *are* ways to effectively express your anger without going completely ballistic.

The next time you feel angry, try to consciously identify the underlying cause. Once you've slowed down enough to do this, simply state out loud to yourself or to whoever is listening, "I'm really angry right now." Then say why you feel angry. For instance, "I'm really angry because I want to be able to drive my kids to their soccer game, instead of having to ask my neighbor to do it."

By taking the time to ask, "What am I really angry about?" you can more clearly recognize the source of your anger. When you can articulate why you're angry, you're less likely to inappropriately or carelessly vent, which can often make things worse.

Many of us have been taught that anger is bad—this is especially true of women. However, anger is not always a negative emotion. When seen from a different perspective, anger can be our ally. In *The Dance of Anger*, Harriet Lerner shines a positive light on anger: "Anger is a signal and one worth listening to. Our anger may be a signal that we are doing more and giving more than we can comfortably do or give. Or, our anger may be warning us that others are doing too much for us, at the expense of our own competence and growth. Our anger can motivate us to say 'no' to the ways we are defined by others and 'yes' to the dictates of our inner self." When seen this way, anger can be viewed as a powerful tool during certain times in our life.

In order to use anger constructively, Dr. Lerner suggests that you routinely ask yourself the following questions when you feel like you might be ready to blow a gasket:

What is it about this specific situation that makes me angry?

What is the real issue?

What do I think and feel?

What do I want to accomplish?

Who is responsible for what?

What do I want to change?

What are the things I am willing to do and not do?

By asking these questions, you're training yourself to clarify your own thoughts so that you can make conscious choices about how you respond to a given situation. This allows you to regain control when you feel like you're losing it. Again, you can use your journal to record your answers.

Knowing your hot buttons can also be an advantage. Many of my clients have learned to identify when they're most likely to lose their temper. Ellen, an MS patient and young mother, says, "I know that when I'm exhausted, I just lose it. My kids come in and they want my attention when I'm trying to make dinner, and tempers flare. It's all I can do to get through the next 30 minutes and put food on the table. I get short because I just need to focus on the task at hand, so I yell and tell them to go into the other room. It makes me feel like an awful Mom, an awful person."

After Ellen identified dinnertime as her most vulnerable period of the day, she put together a plan. She asked the kids to take that time to play outside or watch cartoons. She also started buying prepared foods from the natural food store down the road and using paper plates a few nights a week. Ellen saw that when she was tired she was unable to tend to more than one thing at a time. This made her more likely to lash out in order to get immediate relief from whatever was causing her to feel over stimulated. Now, she tries to minimize how often that might happen by taking back some degree of control over her environment.

Most people are going to have a shorter fuse when they're tired, hot, hungry, or feeling overstimulated. People with MS are especially vulnerable to these triggers. It's our responsibility to exert control over whatever we can, in order to avoid reaching our breaking point. If you're tired, try to make time to rest. If you're hungry, eat (for example, many people find it helpful to eat a wholesome snack *before* cooking dinner). If the music or TV is bothering you, turn it down, go into another room, or wear headphones. If you're overheated, put ice on your neck and wrists. By avoiding reaching these extremes, you will be less likely to act in a way that you might regret later.

Occasionally, we are just pissed off at our disease. This is when we need to say to ourselves or others, "I'm angry at this disease right now, not you." Speaking those few words can bring tremendous relief and understanding.

The Blame Game

Many people with MS can get caught up in the cycle of guilt and self-blame. It's difficult not to feel that you're letting down those you love when you're no longer physically able to meet the needs of others, much less yourself. Patients often feel guilty for simply having MS. This is as rational as feeling guilty for being born, but it is a common response nonetheless.

Those of us with MS frequently feel conflicted about what we would *like* to do for our loved ones and what we are *able* to do. We want to feel productive, we want to do our fair share, and we want to contribute—but often we're limited by what our bodies will allow us to do. The fact that many MS symptoms are transient and invisible compounds this dilemma. Others forget, or are unaware, that we're restricted by our bodies, not by a lack of desire to do more.

Lisa, a thirty-something woman with MS, explains:

> One day it was sweltering hot. I physically crumble in the heat, so my elderly mother had to go get the car and pick me up at the entrance of her air-conditioned assisted living facility. Other elderly residents in the lobby were giving me the evil eye. Here I was, this seemingly young, strong, healthy woman making her mother cart her around like a princess. I wanted to shout to the whole lot of them, "I have MS and I can't get overheated or I get seriously ill!" Instead, I sheepishly dashed out to the waiting air-conditioned car, feeling embarrassed and ashamed.

Sue, a client who decided not to have children because stress and fatigue exacerbate her symptoms, says, "I have good friends, who have a three-year-old and a six-year-old, who want to come and stay with me for a vacation. These are people who would do anything for me. They have opened up their home to me in the past. How can I tell them that the kids will wear me out within two hours? Yet, if I'm not honest, the entire visit will be ruined. I know, because I've tried having kids as houseguests in the past and I ended up in bed for several days."

Can you relate? How many times have you felt guilt and shame because you were unable to function the way a "normal" person would? The way *you* normally would if you didn't have MS? During these times you need to tell yourself, "But I do have MS, and feeling guilty is not supporting me emotionally or physically."

There is no way to have this disease and not feel wracked by guilt, at least occasionally. The important thing is to avoid getting stuck in self-blame that tears down your sense of self-worth. The following section presents some strategies to help minimize the cycle of guilt that MS can create.

Minimizing Guilt

Be honest with yourself. Know your limitations and take them into consideration when committing yourself to social events or other obligations. If you don't overcommit yourself, you will be less likely to let others down.

Be direct. Let people know what your limitations are. For instance, explain to someone looking for help with their children that you would love to baby-sit, but you can only do it for two hours before you begin to get worn out.

Move beyond the superficial. Remember that you're valued by loved ones because of who you are, not because of what you are able to do for them.

Recognize the cycle of guilt as soon as possible. Ask yourself, "What am I feeling guilty about? Is it within my power to change?" If the answer is "Yes," then you must take responsibility, seek to understand why you did what you did, acknowledge to the wronged party what you've done, and make amends. If the answer is "No," you must let the guilt go. Either way, you will be released from the negative impact and the emotional drain that guilt can cause.

The question of guilt always comes back to responsibility. You're not responsible for getting MS. You are responsible for taking care of yourself. You're not responsible for being too tired to entertain. You are responsible for letting your loved ones know what you can and can't do at any given time—for example, when you don't feel up to cooking for the family. Guilt often comes into play when we fail to communicate with others about what we can or cannot do.

Lenor was an engineer who took great pride in her work and her ability to help support her family financially. At the age of 47, Lenor was no longer able to continue her job, due to cognitive difficulties. She explains, "I feel like I'm letting my family down. It kills me to have to leave a job that I love, but the guilt over feeling like I'm not pulling my weight is worse." Lenor had to come to terms with the fact that she didn't choose to leave her job. She didn't choose to get MS. She wasn't choosing to do this to her family and therefore, she wasn't responsible or guilty. Once she was able to accept this reality, she started to focus on ways that she could continue to help her family that didn't involve making money.

Sadness Is Not Depression

In addition to fear, anger, loneliness, and guilt, sadness is another prevalent emotion among MS patients.

Everyone experiences sadness at one time or another. Unlike depression, which can become a chronic debilitating condition, sadness is a temporary state that one passes through. (Since depression is so prevalent in MS patients, I've dedicated the next chapter to depression, its effects and its treatments.)

Sadness is necessary for growth and maturity. It's what we feel when we suffer a loss or experience a tragedy. Our heart aches, our chest may get tight, tears well up in our eyes, and we may feel the need to release the emotion by crying or talking or writing. For the most part, sadness is an appropriate reaction in proportion to the event that is occurring at the moment.

You can expect to feel saddened by the effects of MS. On those occasions when symptoms flare up and you're forced to adapt yet again, you will probably go through a few discouraging days. It's best not to ignore your sadness. Let yourself feel it. Let yourself cry. Acknowledge why you're sad and what you're sad about. Tell someone you love what is making you blue. Spoil yourself for a day or two. Stay in bed, watch TV, read an enthralling novel, pet your dog, allow yourself to wallow in your sadness. It's entirely acceptable to go through this once in a while. The best way to deal with sadness is to simply experience it.

If what you're feeling is sadness rather than depression, your spirits should return to normal within a few days and you will feel like yourself again. Soon you will find that you are taking an interest in others and moving back toward an active, engaging life.

Can Thinking Make It So?

Our mind is a powerful tool that we can use to influence our emotions. Over the years, scientific research has shown that our thoughts do, in fact, sway our feelings. Consider this example: One person is given the diagnosis of MS, and her first thoughts are, "This is terrible, but I'll cope. I know that I have the inner resources to deal with this and that the people in my life will stand by me." Another person thinks, "This is terrible. I don't think I can deal with this. I'm not going to be able to cope and everyone I love will abandon me." The first person's positive thought pattern will greatly reduce her anxiety and fear. The second person will have a much harder time managing her emotional reaction to the disease.

These two people are in the same situation, but their thoughts strongly influence how they handle the information and their emotions. We can use our minds to create positive thoughts that will in turn support our health. This is not the same as stuffing or denying emotions (as was the case with Niki, whose story was told in Chapter 3). When we stuff our feelings, we are becoming unconscious.

When we use our thoughts to lift ourselves up, we're consciously choosing to acknowledge how we feel, and we're taking a proactive step toward feeling better.

Conversely, destructive emotions are often caused by cognitive distortions or negative thoughts. This happens when our way of perceiving reality is skewed by thought patterns that we have developed over the course of our life.

By learning to accurately identify the ways in which your thinking negatively impacts your emotions, you can learn to regain a sense of mastery over your mental well-being. Cognitive therapy is a technique pioneered by Dr. David Burns that teaches you how to change your thought patterns to improve your mood. In this section, you will learn how to influence your thought process in a conscious way and, thus, minimize negative thought patterns. Let's start by illustrating some of the more common ways that our thoughts can be used against us. See if you recognize yourself in any of the following destructive thinking patterns:

Black-and-White Thinking: When we see things in terms of absolutes, we miss the shades of gray. Nothing is all bad or all good. We live in a world of degrees: For example, you feel tired one evening, and you tell yourself that you'll never get your energy back again. (This would be like pouring gasoline on the fire and igniting more misery.) A more rational response might be: "I over did things today and I'm *really* tired. If I get some rest, I'm likely to feel better tomorrow—I usually do." Remind yourself that resting is something you *do* have control over. By simply changing the message that you say to yourself, you will improve your mood, and you may even feel more energetic. This type of positive thinking will also help you be more proactive, and in this case, you will likely get to bed earlier.

Exaggeration: This occurs when you focus on something and magnify it until it becomes larger than life: For example, if you make a mistake at work and begin to worry that you are no longer competent to do your job because you have started having cognitive problems. In this instance, you may have done 100 other things right that day, but rather than giving yourself credit for those things, you blow up the mistake that you made until it overshadows all your accomplishments.

Focusing on the Negative: For instance, you might make progress in physical therapy, but continue to compare yourself to what you used to be able to do before you had MS, rather than acknowledging your improvement. By focusing on your past abilities, rather than the improvements you're making now despite your illness, you are negating the positive aspect of your current experience.

Assuming the Worst: I call this type of thinking the hound dog outlook. No matter what the reality of the situation might be, you expect the worst-case scenario to arise. If the weatherman says there is a chance of rain, you cancel your golf game. Unfortunately, assuming the worst often becomes a self-fulfilling prophecy.

"Shoulding" on Yourself: You tell yourself, "I should be able to walk up those stairs." These destructive "should" statements generally only create guilt and anger, rather than motivation and excitement.

The Sorry Syndrome: This is typically a belief that you personally cause everything that goes wrong even when you have no control over events. For instance, you might blame yourself for having MS and apologize frequently for your symptoms or limitations. People who suffer from this syndrome are constantly saying that they're "sorry." When we offer to accept blame for everything, there is always someone around who is happy to pin it on us.

Do you see yourself stuck in any of these counter productive thinking patterns? Most people fall prey to these distortions and negative internal conversations. However, if your perceptions of reality are distorted by these destructive messages, you are likely to make yourself feel worse than you need to. When you have a disease such as MS, you want to avoid additional mental stress in your life. It's critical that you begin to pay attention to the conversation that goes on inside your head and to consciously choose to replace harmful thoughts with helpful ones.

Denny, a 33-year-old man who came to me after living with MS for two years, presents a good example of a distorted, negative thought process. He remarked, "I'm sure that I'm going to lose my job because of this disease." In reality, the disease had in no way impacted Denny's job performance.

Not everyone who has MS views the world pessimistically, but Denny had developed a mental filter that encouraged him to focus on the worst-case scenario no matter what the situation or reality might be. In this case, Denny experienced several types of negative thinking, including black-and-white thinking, exaggeration, assuming the worst, and focusing on the negative.

Denny's self-defeating way of viewing the world started when he was a young boy. He grew up with a father who lived in constant fear of losing his job. His home was filled with a cloud of anxiety and fear of what might happen. Denny was taught to anticipate and expect the worst possible outcome in any situation.

Once we identified the roots of his belief system, Denny was able to re-train his mind to think more positively and productively. As I mentioned earlier, no amount of worrying about how the future will change our destiny will help, so we might as well expect the best. We will feel much better when we do.

For the next week, try the exercise on the next page, "Negative Thoughts and Positive Answers," to help you recognize your negative thought patterns and begin learning new ways of perceiving situations. With practice, you can develop a more realistic and positive view of the world and your place in it.

In the left column, record the "negative thought" that you catch yourself thinking automatically, often out of habit. In the right column, record a "positive answer" to counteract the negative thinking that you've fallen victim to. Doing this exercise will help steer your mind toward a more positive viewpoint.

Try to do this exercise first thing in the morning (as you get ready for the day), again around 3:00 P.M., and then at night before you go to bed. Keep your journal for at least one week. This should provide enough practice to begin changing deeply ingrained critical self-talk habits. Be patient with yourself during this exercise. It took a long time to develop these habits; they won't be easy to break.

The entries below show how the use of the exercise helped Denny; you should write down the negative thoughts and positive answers that relate to your own situation:

NEGATIVE THOUGHTS AND POSITIVE ANSWERS **

Negative thoughts	Positive answers
"I will end up in a wheelchair and not be able to support my family."	Only 25 percent of MS patients end up in wheelchairs.
	I can learn new skills and adapt to my limitations.
	I can plan for the future.
	I can benefit from current drug therapies.
	I will cope with things as they come and not expect the worst.
	I am able to work.

Denny was able to reduce his anxiety by doing this exercise. He benefited from putting the positive answers in writing so he could refer back to them at any time. Most people find comfort and gain a sense of control by learning to reverse negative thought patterns. Notice the difference in how you feel after practicing this exercise. You'll probably find that it is worth the time and effort to minimize negative self-talk. (Quieting the inner critic is a little like turning down the volume on a noisy radio station and turning up your inner cheerleader.) It's actually just as easy to have a positive thought as a negative one. It's a matter of choice and awareness, and these are decisions you are empowered to make. This is an excellent step to take toward improving both your mental and physical health.

Out-of-Control Feelings

There is a small percentage of MS patients, around 10 percent, who experience what is clinically called "pseudo-bulbar affect." This disturbing emotional experience is characterized by uncontrollable crying or laughing that appears to come from out of the blue. These spells of involuntary emotional outbursts are inappropriate to external circumstances and are unrelated to any underlying feelings of sadness or euphoria.

Because these emotional outbursts are so random and uncontrollable, they can cause a great deal of embarrassment and anxiety for the patient and can be extremely upsetting for those who are witnessing the behavior. As with other MS symptoms, early and accurate diagnosis is imperative so that appropriate treatment can be given. Two tests have been designed to help facilitate the diagnosis of PBA (pseudo-bulbar affect). The Pathological Laughing and Crying Scale (PLACS) is based on an interview conducted by a clinician to quantify the degree of laughing and crying episodes, as well as the level of distress following these emotional periods.

The second test is The Center for Neurologic Study-Lability Scale (CNS-LS). This scale is based on the patients' self-reporting of the frequency, intensity, degree of control, and the inappropriateness of the emotional outbursts.

Although the cause of these emotional outbursts is still inconclusive, according to the National Multiple Sclerosis Society, researchers suspect that PBA is associated with diffuse, bilateral, cerebral involvement that interrupts the corticobulbar tracts involved in the control and expression of emotion.

At this time, PBA is treated primarily with antidepressant medications, which can dramatically reduce the frequency of these emotional outbursts.

Understanding how your feelings and thoughts affect you, both emotionally and physically, plays a key role in your ability to live well with MS.

chapter
five

Treat It and Beat It:
Relieving Depression

*You don't really know how depressed you are until you
start to feel better.*

*— Kathy; age 51, housewife, mother of 3,
MS patient for 10 years*

As a counselor, I'm acutely aware of the tremendous impact depression has on MS patients. Fifty percent of all people with MS will experience a major depressive episode during their lifetime. These are extremely high odds when you consider that only about 10 percent of the rest of the population ever develops depressive symptoms. Although the risk of becoming clinically depressed for those with MS is high, this problem is often undertreated and goes unrecognized by both patients and the medical community. It's vital to be aware that you're susceptible to depression, because too often patients don't realize when they're clinically depressed. As a result, they suffer from a multitude of symptoms needlessly. Most importantly, depression can be life threatening.

According to psychiatrist and MS specialist Dr. Adam Kaplin, it is estimated that up to 25 percent of people living with MS are depressed at any particular time. Suicide is the third leading cause of death among MS patients. These alarming statistics emphasize the need for greater awareness and aggressive treatment of depression among the MS population. Understanding and recognizing depressive symptoms may actually save your life.

Major depression can occur at any time during the disease process and it can be as debilitating as MS itself. In *The Noonday Demon: An Atlas of Depression*, Andrew Solomon aptly describes his experience with depression: "It is too much grief at too slight a cause, pain that takes over from the other emotions and crowds them out. It hurts your heart and lungs. Like physical pain that becomes chronic, it is miserable—not so much because it is intolerable at the moment, as because it is intolerable to have known it in moments gone—and to look forward only to knowing it in the moments to come." If you've experienced the pervasive nature of depression, this quote will ring true.

Since depression is so prevalent in MS patients, and because it is so disruptive and painful for the whole family, this entire chapter is dedicated to the subject.

First, I want to emphasize that once depression is diagnosed, it can usually be effectively treated. Just as advances have been made in treating MS, treatment options for alleviating depression have greatly improved. In the following pages, symptoms and possible treatments for depression are presented.

Causes of Depression in MS Patients

Why is depression so common in MS patients? While it is true that depression can be a direct response to the challenges of living with MS, the issues often goes deeper than that.

1. RESPONDING TO THE DISEASE

Often when patients are first diagnosed, they will go through a period of depression. However, it is essential not to automatically assume that you're depressed simply because you have a chronic illness. You and your doctor should review the many reasons that patients with or without MS are susceptible to depression so that all avenues of appropriate treatment can be explored.

2. DISEASE ACTIVITY

The onset of an exacerbation can be a trigger for depression. Each time an exacerbation occurs following a relatively calm period, many patients go through a wide array of emotions. If you've been in remission and the reality of having the disease has faded, a flare up brings MS back into full focus, making it difficult to deny or ignore. The chronic nature of the disease forces us to continually adjust to its consequences, and this in itself is depressing.

Furthermore, the unpredictable nature of the disease forces us to anticipate future setbacks without a clear idea of what might come next. This unpredictability makes MS unique from most other diseases, which usually have a definitive prognosis and a certain course or outcome. This ambiguity is hard as hell to put up with. Sometimes we simply feel overwhelmed by the challenge of pumping ourselves back up after we have endured an attack or a change in functioning ability. This can trigger periods of depression.

The good news is that with practice and treatment, you can become an expert on how to pull yourself up when you start to go down into that deep, dark pit of despair. In fact, you may even be able to prevent the slide. When you learn what alleviates your depression, you will become more adept at shortening your periods of depression and lessening their impact.

3. CHANGES TO THE BRAIN

Unlike most other chronic conditions, MS can affect the part of the brain that regulates mood. In some cases, depression is thought to be caused by the physiological damage to the central nervous system caused by MS. As nerve damage occurs, depending on the area of the brain that is impacted, moods can become unpredictable. This may explain why depression is more common among people with MS than it is among patients with other chronic conditions that are equally or more physically disabling.

4. MEDICATION SIDE EFFECTS

It is wonderful to finally have several disease-modifying drugs that can help reduce the impact of MS. Unfortunately, depression may be one of the side effects caused by some of these medications. For example, if you're on one of the beta-interferon drugs, you should be attentive to any signs of depression and discuss them with your treating physician (see the list below).

Steroid treatment can also bring on a bout of depression. However, by working with your doctor, you may be able to counter this effect preemptively by taking other prescriptions to lessen the impact of steroids on your moods. One MS patient reported, "I was really nervous about going on steroids because I'd heard horror stories about how you can become so hyper that they have to scrape you off the ceiling or so down that it takes months to feel like yourself again. My doctor and I talked about my fears and he decided to give me some pills to take the edge off of the treatments. Believe me, I would still prefer to never take steroid treatments again, but the medication made it easier."

At this point, if you're feeling concerned about the possibility of developing depression, please know that the intention here isn't to scare you. Rather, the goal is to arm you with facts so that if ever you're faced with a depressive episode, you can be proactive.

Whether your depression is caused by the effects of MS or in response to it, there are numerous treatment options available to you. In most cases, it is possible to find a combination of therapies that will help keep even the worst depression at bay.

Symptoms of Depression

Naturally, the first step in treating depression is recognizing that you are feeling it. However, this isn't always easy. It can be tricky for MS patients to recognize that they're depressed, because typical MS symptoms, such as fatigue and loss of energy, mimic signs of depression. As mentioned in the previous chapter, clinical depression is different from simply feeling sad. The primary difference is that the major depressive symptoms last much longer than the transient feelings of sadness. Clinical depression is an actual medical diagnosis that includes the following symptoms:

- ❖ Feelings of hopelessness, sadness, and despair

- ❖ Loss of pleasure or interest in most activities

- ❖ Significant weight loss or gain; or an increase or decrease in appetite

- ❖ Persistent sleep problems, either insomnia or excessive sleep

- ❖ Ongoing fatigue and loss of energy

- ❖ Feelings of personal worthlessness

- ❖ Inappropriate and excessive guilt

- ❖ Inability to concentrate or make decisions

- ❖ Observable restlessness or slowed movement

- ❖ Recurrent thoughts of death, violence, or suicide

Often these symptoms impair daily functioning, such as the ability to get up and go to work or care for the children. Simply making a meal or taking a shower can feel like an impossible burden. However, depression occurs across a wide continuum. Depending on the number and severity of symptoms, depression is categorized as mild, moderate, or severe.

If you experience five or more of the 10 signs of depression described above on a daily basis for two weeks or more, you are probably depressed and need treatment. For you to begin the healing process, the first step would be to talk with your doctor about treatment options. Your neurologist(s) should be able to provide referrals to several counselors. Get a few names, just as you would when selecting a doctor. If your doctor does not know any counselors, call your local MS society for a referral (see the Resources section at the back of the book for contact information). In addition to neurologists, local MS societies also usually keep lists of local counselors in your area that have been trained to work with MS patients.

Choosing a Therapist

Getting help for depression is just as important as seeking treatment for your MS. Depression rarely goes away on its own, and it often gets worse without treatment. There is no shame in acknowledging that you have a problem, and the sooner you reach out for professional help the better. I myself sought counseling when I was first diagnosed. Even though I was a therapist, I needed the guidance of someone who could provide me with the objective support and insight that I wasn't able to give myself at that time. Counseling got me through the worst period of adjusting to my diagnosis. Everyone needs help sometimes.

I know it is hard to take this next step. It takes a strong and courageous person to deal with depression but you must push yourself to do it. Call a few therapists and schedule interview appointments. Let the therapist know whether you have insurance and ask if their services are covered by your plan. Make it clear with the therapist that you're viewing this as an initial meeting, so you can to get to know each other and to determine if this is going to be a good fit.

You should interview potential therapists, just as you would when selecting a physician. Questions you might ask include the following:

What experience have you had in treating MS patients with depression?

What is your success rate?

How do you feel about using medications to treat symptoms?

What is your theoretical approach?

Are you available after office hours?

Do you work closely with physicians?

All of these questions will help you get the facts, but it is even more important to check your gut reaction. Do you feel comfortable with this counselor? Do you trust the prospective counselor?

Do they seem to be truly listening to what you're saying? Do they seem to care? Do they understand issues relating to chronic illness? These are internal signals that you should pay close attention to. Your therapist can be one of your most important allies in helping you to manage your life with MS. This is going to be a critical relationship, so you should selectively choose the person to whom you will be entrusting the care of your spirit.

Psychiatrists, social workers, psychologists, psychiatric nurses, and licensed professional counselors are all qualified to treat depression. Ideally, try to find someone who has some training or understanding of MS. Be forewarned, however—this may be difficult if you live in a rural or remote location.

Once a connection is made with the right therapist, you can begin to develop a relationship that will help you feel less alone. Counseling can provide you with a greater understanding of your emotions, where they come from, and how to handle them.

Some MS patients find that although they want and need counseling, the costs are prohibitive. Financial restrictions may prevent some from seeking treatment for their depression. However, affordable options maybe available. Talk with your church, your city or county public health department, your local social service agencies, or your local MS chapter to see if they have programs that offer low-cost counseling. Some therapists charge on a sliding-scale basis, depending on income. If you have Medicare, check to see if you have a mental-health benefit that will pay for therapy.

The Prescription Question

Typically, the optimal treatment for depression is a combination of both counseling and antidepressant medication. In fact, the majority of physicians advocate that drug therapy be combined with some form of counseling. Treating depression with medication alone is never as effective as working in conjunction with a qualified professional counselor.

If your depression is impairing your ability to function at home or work, you may want to consider taking an antidepressant medication. In addition to your neurologist, your counselor should be able to determine if this is the right course of treatment. If your counselor believes that medication is needed, they may consult with your physician or a psychiatrist and request a prescription for an antidepressant on your behalf. Don't be concerned if you don't feel better right away after starting on medication. Most antidepressants take about four weeks to begin having an effect and often the improvement is gradual. If there is no improvement after six weeks, tell your counselor and doctor. Frequently, several drugs need to be tried until the right one is found.

If you're resistant to the idea of taking medication, this is understandable. Often, people are hesitant to take medication to relieve depression. Some view taking antidepressants as a sign of weakness. Others are fearful that the medications will change their personalities or reduce their sex drive. Taking antidepressants is a very personal decision, but you should know the facts. Side effects are no longer the issue they once were. The newer drugs are much less likely to cause unpleasant symptoms. If you do experience unwanted effects, again, you can discuss it with your doctor and your counselor. Often, the drug or dosage can be adjusted to make the treatment more tolerable.

There is nothing more discouraging than seeing a patient who really needs medication, but who won't take it because they feel ashamed. It's frustrating that this society still stigmatizes mental illness, but it does. Many have been influenced by this stigmatization and that can make it difficult to accept appropriate treatment. However, taking medication for the medical disease of depression is just as valid as taking medication for your MS.

It's important to note that 80 percent of patients are responsive to medication, but only 50 percent are responsive to their first prescriptive medication. Therefore, do not get discouraged if you have to experiment to get it right. Typically, the more depressive episodes you have, the more likely you are to have subsequent episodes. In general, the episodes that occur over a lifetime become worse and closer together. Taking antidepressants can help to stop this vicious cycle. There is no stronger argument for taking antidepressant medications. Seeking treatment can be difficult, but living with depression is always harder.

Stories of Healing

Over the years, I've treated hundreds of MS patients for depression, and the majority of them found some relief from their symptoms. The following client stories illustrate the various degrees of depression, as well as treatment strategies that were used to bring them relief.

Janet

Janet, a 25-year-old professional, came to me a year after being diagnosed with MS. Having only recently moved out of her parents' home, Janet had fallen into a serious depression. Living on her own for the first time in her life, she'd become extremely isolated. By the time Janet began counseling, she had lost 15 pounds, as well as her interest in going out with friends. Her apartment was a mess because she couldn't find the energy to clean. When she started to miss work because it was too difficult to get out of bed, Janet's parents intervened and insisted that she get some counseling.

Since Janet initially believed that her depressive symptoms were actually caused by the MS symptom of fatigue, this made if difficult for her to recognize that she was depressed. However, because the changes in her behavior had occurred in relation to a specific event (moving out on her own), she was able to accept that she was suffering from a depressive episode. In addition, a number of her symptoms met the criteria for depression.

Although Janet was depressed, she was not suicidal and was willing to come to therapy. After a thorough assessment, I recommended that she talk with her doctor and get a prescription for an antidepressant medication, and continue our weekly counseling sessions. We agreed that if she didn't see improvement over the next three months we would re-evaluate the treatment plan.

During those three months, a low dose of antidepressant medication helped Janet. It allowed her to feel motivated enough to go to work and come to her therapy appointments. We addressed her concerns about MS, as well as her fears of being on her own and meeting new people. Janet had many questions about dating while having MS and how much she should tell her friends and employer about her disease. She'd previously been living in a safe cocoon within her family since her diagnosis and was unsure about how to go forward in her new life while incorporating MS into the picture. Her coping mechanism was avoidance.

By breaking her tasks down into small manageable steps and reaching out for help from others, Janet began to emerge from the fog of depression and to gain a clearer vision of who she truly was. She came to see herself as a capable adult living on her own, facing the same challenges that many of her peers face—with MS as an additional challenge, making her life a bit more complicated.

Within six months, Janet was starting to meet new people in her apartment complex, she was getting to work regularly, and she had started a new exercise program that was helping her regain her appetite and build up her strength. She had even met "a cute new guy" at the gym.

In short, Janet suffered from a moderate degree of depression that was successfully treated with psychotherapy and anti-depression medication.

Mark

Mark is a 55-year-old man who had been living with chronic, progressive MS for two years at the time of our acquaintance. His major complaint was that he no longer enjoyed life. Mark reported, "Everything seems colorless to me. I'm just getting through the days and sleeping through the nights. I'm not even afraid of the future anymore, because I just don't care." Mark's MS had progressed to the point that he was bedridden most of the day. He had paid caregivers with him while his wife was away at work. He had simply withdrawn inside himself and shut out the world. Mark commented, "I used to look forward to my wife coming home, but now, I hardly notice. Food is tasteless, conversation is a great effort. I feel like I just exist." During an extensive assessment, I determined that although Mark was severely depressed, he was not actively suicidal. However, he did have thoughts of death and at times felt his family would be better off without him. I advised Mark to meet with a psychiatrist to review all his medications, since he was on a complicated prescription regime. The psychiatrist made several medication adjustments, which included adding an antidepressant and an anti-anxiety medication to Mark's daily medical-management program.

In addition to meeting with me twice a week, I referred Mark and his wife to a family therapist in order to address the many issues that were affecting them as a couple.

During his course of treatment, Mark did a great deal of work acknowledging his losses. He grieved for the loss of his life before his illness. It was necessary that both he and his wife to talk openly about these changes before they could begin to see how they might find moments of joy in the present.

Mark was able to hear his wife when she told him that it was his smile and warmth and humor that she missed most, not his income or his ability to get around independently. Mark had a significant breakthrough when he realized that the things his wife loved most about him—the essence of who he was—hadn't been taken away by the MS, but by his depressive state, which was something he could work toward changing.

With a combination of counseling and drug therapy, Mark began to reclaim the parts of his old life that were the most meaningful to himself and his wife. Mark remarks, "Before all this happened, I guess I thought I was loved for what I did, not who I was. Now I get it. If I can be a good listener, and be appreciative, and loving toward my wife, that's enough. I can do that."

Once Mark recognized that he still had value despite his illness, his depression began to lift.

Re-creating our self-image and seeing our value in spite of our illness is one of the most powerful weapons we have in keeping depression at bay. In Chapter 7, we will explore self-image and self-esteem in greater depth.

In summary, there is no reason to tolerate depression. If you suspect that you're depressed, I encourage you to take the necessary steps involved in defining your condition and to seek treatment. Your efforts will be rewarded. Poet Jane Kenyon eloquently expresses the promise of relief from depression:

BACK

We try a new drug, a new combination
of drugs and then suddenly
I fall into my life again

like a vole picked up by a storm
then dropped three valleys
and two mountains away from home.

I can find my way back. I know
I will recognize the store
where I used to buy milk and gas.

I remember the house and barn,
and the rake, the blue cups and plates,
and the Russian novels I loved so much,

and the black silk nightgown
that he once thrust
into the toe of my Christmas stocking.

By treating your depression, you, too, will begin to find your way back.

chapter
six

Stress and MS:
How to Soothe Yourself

Stress always invites my MS to come out and play.

— Libby; 27-year-old insurance agent, MS patient for three years

People living with MS intuitively know what the scientific community has just begun to prove—that stress has an impact on our health. I want to be clear that stress does not cause MS but can compromise the body's ability to fight disease. When I give presentations to MS audiences, I always ask, "Who out there has noticed that your health suffers when you are stressed?" Inevitably, 90 percent of the audience will knowingly wave their hands in the air. The other 10 percent are probably just shy. Everyone laughs in recognition. Have you recognized a correlation between feeling stress and your symptoms?

Stress and Your Health

The connection between stress and health is now gaining national attention. For example, a recent issue of *Newsweek* magazine (September 2004) reported that the mind's effect on the body is now the next frontier in scientific research. As we learn to more clearly recognize this connection in our own bodies, we can begin to manage the effects that stress has on our symptoms. Once our awareness becomes focused on how our body reacts to stress, we can respond to it more proactively.

Clients frequently report instances in which stress seems to trigger symptoms. Sara, a 46-year-old MS patient, remarked:

> I was planning my wedding before I knew that I had MS. I was 25 years old and had the world by the tail. It was an exciting time in my life. I loved my fiancé and felt really good about getting married, but the details of the wedding were totally stressing me out. Deciding on a dress and trying to lose weight, making all the choices (a band, who to invite, what to serve, the right photographer), and trying to work at the same time, it was intense. Then one morning before the wedding, I woke up and the right side of my face was numb. I could feel my skin if I touched it, but it was like I'd been to the dentist and he had pumped my face full of Novocain. I could smile, but it didn't feel like I was smiling. I went to my general practitioner and he said it was probably a virus called Bell's palsy and that it would pass. This calmed me down a bit, but I still felt so weird during all the wedding photo sessions. I thought my face looked distorted. When I see those pictures now, 20 years later, I realize they reflect my first MS attack. I'm convinced that the stress of the wedding brought it on.

Stories like Sara's clearly imply a relationship between stress and symptoms.

Stress is part of life for everyone, but frequent stress is another matter. Over time, chronic stress takes its toll on the body and can cause impaired memory, a weakened immune system, high blood pressure, headaches, skin problems, and a host of other things that you would rather avoid.

The federal government will spend $16 million on mind-body research in 2006 to better understand how feelings and thoughts affect our health. Current research already shows that physiological states or "feeling states" affect our health just as directly as our physical condition. In fact, experts report that 60 to 90 percent of doctor visits involve stress-related complaints.

The reason stress plays such an important role in our physical well-being takes some further explanation. The fight-or-flight response that we've inherited from our hunter-gatherer ancestors helps us respond to perceived danger or threats.

When we feel scared or stressed, we produce adrenaline. This creates that rush of sensations you feel when you just barely avoid a car accident or are waiting to get potentially scary news from your doctor. Your heart starts pounding, your hands sweat, and you feel lightheaded; this is the classic full-blown stress response.

This surge of energy can be helpful when you need to run for your life, but your body does not know the difference between being chased by a predator and having to take a shot each week to treat your MS. It just experiences stress.

When we're under stress, the body focuses all its resources in our defense, pumping blood to our arms and legs so we can respond effectively—fight or flee. In order to achieve this preparation level, functions such as the immune response and digestion are temporarily inactivated. (You may have experienced this personally—have you ever noticed how easily you caught cold during a hectic or stressful time in your life, such as during school finals or when you were under work deadlines?)

Given this inherited tendency to fight or flee, a range of situations can set off a stress reaction, even something as benign as buying a car. Beth, an MS sufferer and 33-year-old mother of two, tells the following story:

> I was buying my first "new" used car. I'd never negotiated for a large purchase like that before and, of course, I'd heard all the scary stories about how used-car dealers will try to rip you off. I went *into* the dealership feeling defensive. I found the car I just had to have and the negotiations started. The salesman kept leaving me in his office to go check in the back with his manager and see if he could meet my offer. Each time he came back, we had to dicker again. I was getting both angry and

stressed. I felt really conflicted because I didn't want to leave without that car. Well, this went on for a while and, sure enough, my legs started to go numb and my foot-drop came back. Then I started to become stressed out about my symptoms, so I finally caved in, paid for the car, and left.

Beth's story not only points out how our *reactions to our symptoms* can make the situation worse. This can be a real catch-22. Because MS symptoms can come on so suddenly, patients tend to panic when they begin to feel old familiar problems crop up or new symptoms emerge. Unfortunately, panicking only makes the symptoms more noticeable and aggravating.

In addition to facing normal everyday stresses and wrestling with symptoms, MS patients have to deal with the incredible pressures that are caused by the disease itself. MS affects many different parts of life, from cognitive functioning to sexual functioning, from friendships to parenting, and from housework to careers. Everything is impacted by MS, and almost everything is made more stressful by it.

With all of these challenges, you obviously can't completely eliminate stress from your life. No one can. Over the years, you will continue to face both good and bad stresses. Babies will be born, loved ones will die, your health will ebb and flow, and some of your dreams will come true and others will slip by. This is life. You're here to experience all of it. However, *how* you experience it will have a dramatic impact on the quality of your life. Since you have MS and stress can aggravate it, you have a greater responsibility than the average person to learn how to respond to stress creatively and proactively, rather than simply reacting to it. Your health and happiness are at stake, as is the well-being of your loved ones.

Although we cannot avoid stress, there are strategies you can adopt to manage it. We know from research that once the stress response is triggered, the immune system only reactivates once the threat of danger has passed. The restorative period following stress is described as the relaxation response. Using this knowledge, anyone who practices the stress reducing techniques in this chapter will find that they can improve the way they experience stress and obtain the ability to access the relaxation response on command.

What Can We Control?

One day, Kathy came through my office door. Although she had successfully managed to adapt to her MS over the past 20 years, she was going through an incredibly difficult time in her life, and as a result her symptoms were worsening. During our first session, she told her story: "I don't know where to begin, but I guess it will just come out the way it's supposed to. My husband lost his job. My mother has been diagnosed with Alzheimer's disease. Dad has terminal cancer and my daughter, who also has MS, was just hospitalized. I've always been able to handle things; I guess because they mainly impacted me, but now I think I'm losing it."

Of course, Kathy thought she was going crazy. She felt as if she'd lost control over everything she cared about in the world. Since we couldn't change the facts of Kathy's situation, we started to work on how she handled her stress. She had to find relief fast.

Once Kathy realized that the only thing she *did* have control over was how she responded to the stresses in her life, she started to make positive choices. The first step was letting go of the idea that all her worrying over the people she loved was going to solve any problems. She recognized that by worrying she was wasting precious energy that was needed to take care of herself and her family. Kathy said that worrying was a habit for her. She admitted that worrying made her feel as if she had some control over the outcome of events. As we reviewed her false reasoning, Kathy conceded that worrying had never changed the course of things in the past and most likely it wouldn't in the future. Acknowledging this allowed Kathy to start working on what she *could* do to make things better in her life.

Next, we broke down Kathy's concerns into manageable increments and addressed each issue one at a time. For instance, since Kathy's husband was not working, she asked him to stay with their daughter at the hospital during the day. This allowed Kathy to focus her attention on her parents. Together, we did some research and located an adult day-care center that her mother could go to for up to eight hours a day, five days a week. Since her father's cancer was terminal, Kathy was able to get an order from his doctor for hospice care. The hospice staff was able to visit her father in his home and they provided a great deal of comfort to all the family members. Kathy also spoke with her father about some of her financial concerns, and he was able to lend her some money to ease that worry. After marshalling together all these resources, Kathy felt empowered and realized she was supported by others. She was now putting her energies into problem solving rather than simply passively worrying, and this gave her strength. Once Kathy had identified what she could control and had a plan in place, her stress abated.

What We Can't Control

Most MS patients live with a lot of stress. The very nature of the disease is stressful. Since no doctor can accurately forecast our medical future, we're left to wonder, "How sick will I get?" We can feel extremely powerless. I've actually had a client tell me that he'd rather have gotten a terminal disease than MS, because at least then he would know what to expect and would no longer have to live with the uncertainty of a disease like MS. That client came to terms with his illness and changed his mind eventually, but his attitude shows how much anxiety can be involved in living without answers. It's easy to stress out over the unknown and things that we can't control, but this gets us nowhere fast.

The next time you feel stressed ask, "Is this something I have any control over?" If the answer is "Yes," then take whatever action is required to relieve the stress, but if the answer is "No," then let the stress go. Just give it up.

Living by the words of the serenity prayer is a great way to let go of the things we can't control and, in turn, let go of stress. When you find yourself getting carried away by stress, just say out loud, "God, grant me the serenity to accept the things I cannot change, the courage to change the things I can, and the wisdom to know the difference."

Stress-Reduction Practices

So far you've learned that managing stress and worry can improve your health. Now it is time to learn some stress-management practices. The following stress-reducing techniques are tried and true. They've helped millions of people cope with the stress in their lives. I urge you to give them a try.

MEDITATION

When you feel at peace, nothing can harm you. But how do you achieve peace when you're in pain, anxious, blue, or exhausted? Many people have discovered meditation to be the answer. Not long ago, meditation was viewed as an alternative form of healing or spiritual practice, but recently it has been gaining credibility in the scientific community. The National Institutes of Health has put 2.1 million dollars into research to compare the positive effects of meditation against the benefits of antidepressants and other prescription drugs. Medical clinics across the country are offering meditation classes to help patients reduce pain and anxiety. Often the patients who are "untreatable" or who don't benefit from conventional medicine seek out meditation as a last resort with surprisingly effective results. This ancient tradition is becoming more mainstream, and the primary reason is that people are experiencing calming and physical benefits from practicing meditation.

To put it simply, meditation is a way of training your mind. Just as we can train our muscles to lift weights, we can train our mind to focus on thoughts that will have a positive effect and to let go of thoughts that are destructive. The following steps will help you get started with a meditation program:

❖ Set aside at least 20 minutes each day to practice. You can start with just five minutes a day, but research shows that a 20-minute session is needed to experience the full benefits of meditating. Practicing 20 minutes, twice a day, is optimal.

❖ Make sure you won't be interrupted. Turn off the phone and let family members know that this is your time. Unless someone is actually bleeding, they need to give you some peace and quiet.

❖ Set a timer or an alarm clock to go off in 20 minutes so that you don't have to be distracted by watching the time.

❖ If you're able, sit in a comfortable position. Lying down is discouraged, but if that's the only position you can tolerate, then it will work.

❖ Close your eyes and take a few deep, full breaths. Pay attention to your physical body and how it feels against the floor or chair and in your clothes.

❖ Now focus on your breath and nothing else. As thoughts come into your head, notice them and then bring your attention back to the breath. The goal isn't to completely avoid intrusive thoughts, but to notice it when you do have them and then go back to the breath. It doesn't matter if you have 100 thoughts in one minute (many of us do); as long as you bring your consciousness back to your breath, you've been successful.

❖ Once the alarm goes off, you can open your eyes and bring your awareness back to the room.

❖ Do this exercise twice every day.

This is a very basic introduction to meditation; however, there are many good books and classes, which go into greater detail, available to help you learn how to meditate. You may find it helpful to begin with a book that provides a good overview of resources for stress reduction, such as *Full Catastrophe Living* by Jon Kabat-Zinn. This and other useful books and tapes are listed in the Resources section of this book. Many gyms and hospitals also teach meditation or stress reduction classes. Group meditation can be a wonderful opportunity to become familiar with these techniques. A class setting gives you the chance to ask questions and talk with others who are interested in the discipline.

Mary, a vibrant woman in her thirties, came to see me after living with the diagnosis of MS for about a year. Although the physical impact of MS was minor for her, causing numbness and occasional fatigue, the psychological pressure of having MS had taken over her thoughts. She constantly worried about what might happen to her. After learning how to meditate and practicing 20 minutes a day for three months, Mary said, "MS no longer has control over me. I realize I can direct my own thoughts and I don't have to give all my attention and energy to the disease if I don't want to." By learning how to train her mind to focus on a single thing, like breathing, Mary was able shift her thoughts when she found herself going into the land of "what ifs."

EXERCISE

Physical exercise is another extremely effective stress-management technique. If you could take a pill that would help you lose weight, make life more interesting, introduce you to other people, build confidence, reduce stress, and take the focus off MS for a while, would you ask your doctor for a prescription? Of course you would! If there were a pill that could do all that, we would all be popping it like M & Ms.

Well, the prescription you're looking for doesn't come in a pill; it comes in the form of exercise. Too often people with MS feel that their physical limitations prevent them from exercising. However, by working with a physical therapist and being creative, most people with MS are able to do some type of exercise to get their blood pumping and their muscles moving.

Heather, a woman in her late fifties who had been living with MS for more than 15 years, could barely walk without using two canes, but when she went to her water aerobics class, she floated with the best of them. Her class not only helped her keep some of her muscle tone, it also gave her a wealth of emotional and social support. Most people in her class had some type of physical limitation and they were able to encourage and inspire each other to stay active, no matter what.

Using your body helps to let off steam and release stress and anxiety. Exercise can also help you sleep better, feel less irritable, give you more energy, and make you stronger. Find 30 minutes a day to exercise, do something you really enjoy, and preferably do it with a family member or friend.

If you find that your symptoms are aggravated by heat, you may want to explore purchasing some of the cooling products specifically designed to keep your temperature down while you exercise. You can find suppliers listed in the Resources section.

Check with your doctor and get clearance before you start an exercise program. If you feel stymied because of physical limitations, ask your doctor to write you a prescription for a few sessions with a physical therapist. A therapist's expertise should help you tailor a program that will meet your needs and get you started.

YOGA

Recently, researchers have found that yoga practice has many benefits for MS patients. Oregon Health Sciences University recently reported that participants who went through a six-month yoga program had an increase in energy and stamina, as well as improved flexibility and balance.

Yoga is very popular these days. Once viewed as a mystical or religious practice, yoga has become more accessible now that gyms and community centers have begun to offer classes. Most people find that they are able to easily perform the beginner yoga poses.

The beauty of yoga is that you're encouraged to go at your own pace, not comparing yourself to anyone else, but simply trying to stretch your own limits in a gentle, forgiving way. Most classes end with a brief meditation as well, so you get the added benefit of winding down and getting centered before you complete your session. Classes typically last about an hour. Many of my clients report enjoying classes in the morning or the middle of the day, before fatigue sets in.

If getting to class is difficult for you, try purchasing one of the following videos, or better yet, visit your local library and borrow any available introductory yoga tapes.

Accessible Yoga for Every Body is a great beginner tape for those who are a little less flexible or for those who just want to go slow. *Power Yoga Total Body*, with instructor Rodney Yee, who happens to be very easy on the eyes, is a good tape for those who want more of a challenge. Video suppliers are listed in the Resources section.

PROGRESSIVE RELAXATION

When all you really feel like doing is lying down, progressive relaxation exercises are a great option. This stress reducer should be practiced in a quiet environment where you can spread out and insure that you won't be disturbed. Once you've banned family members from entering the room and turned off the phone, follow these guidelines:

❖ Lie down in a comfortable position; be sure you're warm.

❖ Begin by taking a few full, deep breaths and just focus on your breathing.

❖ Once you begin to relax, focus on your toes and breathe into them. Once you're conscious of your toes and how they feel in your socks, curl them under your feet and squeeze them tight, hold that for just a few seconds, and then relax them. Just let them go and draw your breath back down into your toes.

❖ Next, flex your feet up and hold for a second. Then relax and breathe into your ankles.

❖ Then move on to the calves and tighten your calve muscles. Hold for a few seconds, and then release. Feel the relaxation sensation in your calves once you stop contracting the muscle.

❖ Next move to your buttocks. Squeeze your buttocks and hold for a second, then release. Feel your entire lower body relax.

❖ Then tighten your stomach. Hold for a few seconds and then relax. Breathe out through your stomach, and on the following in breath, imagine warm air relaxing your stomach.

❖ Now move to your chest and upper body. Tighten your chest muscles, and then let go. Breathe out and let your chest relax and collapse.

❖ The arms are tightened next. Try to make a fist and flex your arm muscles, and then release your hands and arms, letting the relaxation wash over you.

❖ Finally, tense your face by making a grimace. Feel the tension in your face, and then release it.

❖ Conclude by imagining that you are taking in a warm ray of light in through the top of your head and letting the light enter all of your body, warming you and relaxing you throughout your entire body. Take a few more deep breaths. Now open your eyes and slowly bring your focus back to your surroundings.

If you have trouble sleeping, as many people with MS do, this can be a good exercise to practice prior to falling asleep. Relaxing your entire body helps you to calm down and transition from wakefulness to sleep. If you make time for this exercise during the day, you may want to take a nap or leave yourself time afterward to become alert again. A progressive relaxation exercise is also included in the Jon Kabat-Zinn *Mindfulness Meditation* tape.

GUIDED IMAGERY

Guided imagery is a wonderful skill that allows you to create an altered state where you can set a scene and influence your mind and your mood by using your imagination.

Studies show that using guided imagery can improve the immune system, speed healing, and reduce pain. When using guided imagery with my clients, I find that they're able to become calm and centered even in the midst of very stressful situations. It comes as no surprise that the more we feel we're in control of our emotional state, the less anxious we become and the better we feel about ourselves. Using guided imagery can give you a sense of mastery over your environment, your stress level, and your thinking.

Initially, some people are fearful of using guided imagery as a relaxation tool. You may be afraid that you will somehow lose control. In reality, you're taking control when you go into an altered state because you're creating your own reality. Once you experience the effects of guided imagery, you will appreciate the positive results it offers.

The following instructions take you through a very basic imagery exercise. It's best to do this exercise twice a day for three weeks before deciding whether or not it is helpful in reducing stress, because it can take practice to develop the skills required to really go into a deep relaxed state. You may want to read the script I've provided into a tape recorder and then play it back to yourself. Or you can purchase a guided imagery tape and play it. Ordering information for tapes can be found in the Resources section at the back of this book.

Go to a quiet room where you won't be disturbed. Turn down the lights and turn off the phone. Put on some relaxing music if you like. Sit or lie in a position that allows your back to be aligned and straight. Begin by taking a few deep, relaxing breaths to set the tone and mood.

Sample Script

Take a deep, full, relaxing breath and then release the breath. Visualize any unhealthy energy leaving your body with the exhale. Then envision breathing clean, healthy energy and healing light deep into your lungs. Do this two or three times, at your own pace. Follow the natural flow of your breath. Feel the breath enter your body and notice how it relaxes you more each time you inhale and exhale. Notice how your stomach expands with each inhalation and deflates with each exhalation. Keep your attention on your breath, and now imagine that you are focusing it to soothe any constricted areas in your body.

Send the breath to the places that are sore, or in spasm, or tight—and feel the breath surround those areas and loosen the tension. With each breath, imagine that you are exhaling pain and tension and inhaling comfort and relaxation. The tense spots are releasing and you are relaxing your entire body. You are becoming as relaxed and loose as jello and this is a comforting feeling.

If your thoughts turn away from your breath, gently recognize them, give them a nod, and let them go on their way. These thoughts can be attended to later, but for now, send them away with your out-breath and breath in clear, empty space so that your mind can rest for a while.

If any intrusive feelings arise, acknowledge them and assure them that you will get back to them later and then send those away with your out-breath, as well. Breathe in calm, clean, peaceful feelings for just these few moments.

Next, envision yourself walking up a flight of stairs. There are five steps in front of you. As you walk up the first step, you become calmer and more relaxed. On the second step, you go deeper into relaxation and peace. On the third step, you notice that your body is completely relaxed. On the fourth step, you are so relaxed you feel as if you are almost floating. On the fifth step, you are totally relaxed and curious about the door that appears in front of you. You know that once you open that door, you will walk into a space that is safe and welcoming and familiar.

As you turn the doorknob and push the door open, you see a place that you have always dreamed of. At first, you smell your favorite fragrance and it is calming and relaxing; it might be vanilla or jasmine or cinnamon rolls, but the smell is very real and very welcoming. The scent draws you in and welcomes you.

Next, you look around and see your favorite scene. It might be the ocean or the forest or a favorite room. As you look around you, take in each detail and color and texture. You are surrounded by all the things you love and comforted by this place, knowing that you are where you're supposed to be.

Do you hear the wind or the ocean waves or birds singing or a grandfather clock ticking? Listen carefully to the sounds of this special place. Take in this spot with all your senses and be comforted by its peacefulness.

Inhale the essence of this place and, again, let yourself relax further with each breath, knowing that you are safe and secure and in a place that is peaceful. Here you can let your guard down, you can be yourself, you can move along at your own pace, and you can take the time you need to become centered and feel completely at peace: no worries, no rushing around, no fear... just soothing, relaxing comfort right here and right now, yours to enjoy. And, as you take this place in, know that you can recall this place and this time at any moment. This is your place to return to and enjoy whenever you need a break or feel the need to completely relax.

When you are ready, you can return to the door. As you open the door, turn to bid farewell to your special spot for now. As you step down from the top step, you become a little more aware of the place you are in now. At the fourth step, you notice your body and feel your clothes surrounding your skin. At the third step, you become more aware of your surroundings and more alert. At the second step, you feel the space surrounding you and you hear the sounds of the room you are in now. At the first step, you open your eyes and take in your environment. Very slowly and gently, you can once again focus your attention on the room you are physically in. As you recall your special place, remember that you can return to that spot at any time and recreate this calm feeling whenever you need to relax.

This exercise should only take about 10 minutes. It's best to do it upon waking and before going to sleep because that's when you're most open to entering a relaxed, altered state. It's important that the tape you listen to sounds calming and has imagery that has meaning for you. You can customize a tape for yourself or you can ask someone who has a soothing voice to record a tape for you.

The book *Staying Well with Guided Imagery*, by Belleruth Naparstek, does a great job describing the philosophy and research behind guided imagery. It also gives several script examples and answers commonly asked questions about the practice. You can find where to order her materials in the Resources section.

Guided imagery is an incredibly easy way to manage stress and take a mini mental vacation.

TEAPOT BREATHING

This is one of the most popular exercises I use during my speaking presentations. People love the "teapot" breathing exercise because it is so simple and it engages many of our senses. By using your breath to slow down your heart rate and blood pressure, you can train yourself to become calm in any situation. The beauty of this exercise is that it is always accessible and available. At any given moment, your breath is always available, ready to be used as a tool to soothe you.

This exercise was named for the sound that you make upon releasing your breath. During the exhale, you make a hissing sound similar to the sound steam makes when water has come to a boil in a teapot. The following steps will guide you through the process:

- Sit or lie comfortably and close your eyes.

- Begin by taking a deep, full breath.

- Imagine drawing up cleansing water through the soles of your feet to the top of your head. See your body filling up with the cleansing water as you fill your lungs with air.

- When you have a full breath of air, release the breath at your own pace and make a hissing sound as breath leaves your body.

- Imagine your body releasing any negative emotions with the exhale.

- Repeat this three times.

You may feel a bit dizzy the first few times you try this exercise. Just remember to go at your own pace and take a deep, but comfortable breath. Give yourself a few moments before you stand up.

While doing this exercise, you're engaging your mind. You're asking yourself to use imagery, to breathe, and to make the hissing sound all at once. This will automatically force you to shift your focus and take attention off anything worrisome. It's an effective way to quickly reset your mental attitude.

MASSAGE

Since we usually carry stress in our body, massage can be a wonderful way to release built-up tension. You may want to hire a professional masseuse, but massage is also something that you can do with a loved one. Setting up a weekly ritual at which time you give each other a massage is a perfect way to experience intimacy and to maintain physical contact, especially if MS has inhibited your ability to be sexually intimate. No matter what one's physical limitations, everyone needs physical contact.

Be sure to communicate with whoever gives you a massage. Let them know if their touch is too deep or hurts in any way. A massage should not be painful. Pain causes your body to tense up, which defeats the purpose of a relaxing massage. It's often helpful to stay quiet during a massage and just to focus on the physical sensations. Many people prefer not to talk during a massage, but just relax. This way, you give yourself the gift of receiving pleasure, without having to expend any energy during the process. How often are you able to do that?

Others find that they enjoy talking during the massage. Physical touch can help you to let go of emotions that may have been building up. This can also be a wonderful release. Just check in with yourself prior to your massage and ask yourself what you need at that moment.

THOUGHT CONTAINMENT

Since our thoughts often precede or create stress, it is important to learn ways to curtail negative thinking. We cannot experience a negative emotion without first having a thought that creates the feeling. By using "thought containment," you're able to create a space to allow your thoughts to exist, but you limit the impact they have on you.

For this to be effective, it is important to come up with some type of imagery that has meaning for you. One client I worked with would feel flooded with thoughts before she went to bed. She could not turn off her mind. She decided to use the image of a box to contain her thoughts. At night before she went to sleep, she acknowledged each thought and then mentally put it away in a box. Then she imagined closing the box on her thoughts and putting it under her bed. She told herself they would be there tomorrow if she needed to examine them again. In doing this, she was able to let go of the troubling thoughts that kept her up at night and to embrace a solid night's sleep.

Another way to contain thoughts is to write them down and then let them go. Using your journal, or just keeping a note pad by your bed, can allow you to have a place to put your thoughts so that they can leave you alone for awhile. For many, keeping a journal is very therapeutic. In the process, you may discover a pattern of thinking that seems to have a positive or negative effect on your mood and health. By containing your thoughts, you begin to take control of your mind and, as a result, your outlook will significantly improve.

If you're interested in learning more about how your thoughts impact your feelings, read *Feeling Good*, by David Burns, M.D. This book goes into great detail about the mind-body connection and how feelings follow thought. In addition, you might want to review Chapter 4 of this book, especially the section "Can Thinking Make It So?"

HAVE FUN

The truth is, between treatments, physical therapy, doctor appointments, and other MS demands, it is tempting to become absorbed with your disease. It's easy to make MS the focus of your life, and this is a natural response to the initial diagnosis or during exacerbations—but try not to give MS more attention than it deserves. Maintaining a balance between your disease and the rest of your life is essential.

The chronic nature of MS forces us to live with illness for many years; you might as well endeavor to enjoy yourself as much as you can during the journey. Having fun is like sticking your tongue out at your disease. You may have to work a little harder to find the joys and pleasures that life has to offer you, but if you search, they will appear.

Can you remember one thing that made you happy when you were a kid? Perhaps it was sailing or camping or curling up with a good book. Take a moment to identify one activity that used to bring you joy but has long since been abandoned.

For instance, one of my clients loved to sing as a child. She remembered how special it made her feel to be in her church choir. As an adult, she no longer made time for singing. Once she identified that this was something she could still do and enjoy, she took action and joined a choir. Eventually, she even signed up for singing lessons. She describes her experience after bringing song back into her life: "When I sing, I don't think about having MS. I'm just in the moment, using my talents and having fun. It's a relief to focus on something I do well instead of on my limitations."

When you shift your focus from what you can't do to what you can do, life will always improve. Just because you can't do something the way you used to do it doesn't mean you can't do it at all. It's better to dance for 10 minutes, or golf only nine holes using a cart, than to miss out on a good time.

Doing something that isn't MS-related can be a very important stress-management tool for both for you and your family members. If you brainstorm, perhaps you will come up with something fun that you can all do together.

BIOFEEDBACK

Many people are now using biofeedback as a way to manage stress or pain and to improve their health. Biofeedback teaches you to get more in touch with your body and to control your physical responses and emotions such as anxiety or discomfort. Chances are you've already used biofeedback. If you step on a scale and see you've gained a few pounds and then decide to cut back on sweets until your weight comes back down, you're using biofeedback. You've taken specific feedback about your body and used that information to change your behavior.

However, to take biofeedback a step further, you'd need to find a trained specialist. Your doctor may be able to recommend one. Biofeedback clinicians use electronic equipment that provides feedback to the participant about body signals such as pulse rate, blood pressure, or the degree of muscle tension. For example, most people are surprised to learn that their blood pressure can go up by as much as 20 points when they just talk about a stressful subject. The beauty of the biofeedback equipment is that it can measure your responses in specific, measurable terms. As you learn how to moderate your responses to stress, the feedback you get will reflect that improvement (for example, as a more normal blood pressure reading). This type of information helps patients increase their sensitivity to their own physiological states and bodily reactions.

Biofeedback is usually provided in an office setting, where you are connected to a monitor, with small button-sized sensors that pick up electrical signals from your skin and muscles. The monitor then translates these signals into something tangible such as a flashing light, a soft beeping signal, or a number (for example, your pulse rate). If your goal is to reduce muscle tension, the clinician will teach you how to relax by training you to slow down the flashing or beeping sound with focused intention. The biofeedback technician acts as a coach to help you set goals and shows you how to improve your performance as you learn to take control of your responses.

In addition to learning how to use the signals from the machine to calm yourself, you're taught some form of relaxation exercise, such as one of those previously mentioned in this chapter. You'll also be taught to identify the circumstances that trigger stress or other symptoms and ways to avoid or cope with those stressful events.

According to the National Institute of Mental Health, experts believe that physical responses to stress can become habitual. When the body is repeatedly aroused, feelings of stress can be constantly triggered. Many clinicians find that their clients have forgotten how to relax. Using biofeedback can help you recognize a relaxed state and remember how to re-create it.

One of the most positive aspects of biofeedback is that it puts you back in charge of your body's response to stress. You discover how you're contributing to your own distress, and by realizing this, you may be able to reduce some of your physical symptoms.

Researchers believe that relaxation is one of the key components of these techniques, particularly in disorders that are brought on or made worse by stress. These assumptions are based on what we know about the effects of stress on the body; stressful events produce strong emotions, which arouse physical responses.

If you'd like to learn more about biofeedback, you can locate further information in the Resources section.

Because biofeedback has become a widely accepted technique for treating stress-related problems, your insurance plan may help pay for part of the cost.

⌘ ⌘ ⌘

You've just learned 10 of the most effective relaxation techniques available to help manage stress. I strongly advise that you choose two of these activities and do them every day for 60 days. If you have a loved one or friend who can participate in one of these activities, ask them to join you. It will increase your chances of sticking with the new routine, and the techniques will lower your companion's stress as well.

Sixty-Day Symptom Log **

As they take steps to reduce the stress in their lives, clients find that they have achieved amazing results when they've used the following "Symptom Log" to monitor their MS symptoms. I encourage you to incorporate this tool into your new stress-management regime. It will give structure to your stress reduction plan and allow you to monitor your physical improvements. You can use your journal to create your symptom log.

STEP ONE

Describe any current MS symptoms you're experiencing:

_____

_____

STEP TWO

List the two stress-management activities you plan to introduce into your day and the time of day you will schedule them:

STEP THREE

Write down who you will be doing these activities with and on what days:

DAY: _____ ____

Activities: _____

Completed: Y/N

Partner: _____

Time: _____

Symptoms:

How did you feel after the stress-management exercise?

_____

If you didn't complete a stress-management activity, what got in your way?

_____

_____

Have you noticed any improvement in your symptoms? Yes/No

Make copies of this sheet and use it each day during the 60-day plan to track your results. I highly recommend using the log. It can be hard to notice incremental improvements unless you keep a daily log. The log also helps you identify any obstacles that prevent you from finding time for stress management in your day and it can motivate you to overcome those challenges. Using the "Symptom Log" helps you clearly identify which exercises are the most effective and which you enjoy the most. One client exclaimed, "I feel empowered to help myself by using this log. It's all up to me, and when I see the results, I want to stick with my stress-management program!"

One of the best ways family members and loved ones can support the person with MS in their life is to encourage them to maintain a stress-management program and do one of these exercises with them daily. You will be helping to improve the quality of your loved one's life, as well as your own.

Identifying Triggers

Ironically, hearing that we should avoid stress can actually add to our feelings of anxiety because we know it is impossible to eliminate stress completely from our lives. Our only realistic option is to learn how to manage it effectively. In addition to stress management techniques, another way for us to do this is by paying attention to what events stress us out and by minimizing our exposure to those events.

Because MS affects the central nervous system, triggers such as noise, movement, or crowds can have a huge impact on our energy level and make us more susceptible to experiencing stress. A simple activity like going to the mall for a few hours can leave us feeling shell-shocked. Trish, an MS patient and mother of three, realized that every time she came home from a shopping trip she'd feel wiped out and need to crash for several hours afterwards. Once Trish identified going to the mall as a stress trigger, she was able to make different choices that helped her eliminate the stressor. Since shopping was not an activity Trish necessarily loved to do, she learned how to shop on the Internet and saved herself from the dread and exhaustion of trips to the mall. This greatly reduced her stress level.

It is worth mentioning that we are at especially high risk for experiencing stress during the holidays. This is a time of year that is clearly hectic for everyone, but for people with MS it is especially difficult to bounce back from the demands of the season. Over the years, I've seen a distinct pattern of increased exacerbations in clients during December and January, which makes this an especially important time to notice your stress triggers. We can experience very different stress reactions during this time of year depending on what our relationships are like with family members and what expectations we have. Some are energized by the holidays and they enjoy time with family and friends. Others feel overwhelmed by the social commitments and additional demands of the season. Still others react to all the sweet and starchy foods that are part of traditional holiday meals. Many folks find that they can barely get through the festivities and afterward need about three days' bed rest to recover.

As you identify what your holiday stress triggers are, you can reduce your exposure to those triggers. For instance, one client acknowledged that staying at her parents' home during Christmas made her feel as if she had no control over her environment or the amount of rest she could get. So, she decided that when she went to see her family she would stay in a hotel. This gave her a refuge where she could reduce her stimulation and get the rest that she required.

Grocery shopping is another stress trigger. For some, it's a joy to go to the store, but for others making decisions about what to buy and then getting the groceries in and out of the car can feel like a daunting task. In this case, you may ask your spouse or a close friend to do this chore. You can write out the list and have them shop. You may even have an online shopping service or at-home delivery service available in your town.

Stress Journal

The goal of stress management is to begin seeing your situation in a new light. This will enable you to think outside the box and brainstorm about ways that you can reduce your stress triggers. To get a handle on these triggers, try using the following "Stress Journal." This simple tool can be useful whenever you feel stressed out, and it will help you identify the situations that really push you over the edge.

Use the "Stress Journal" along with your "Symptom Log" for 60 days to create an effective stress-management plan customized to your needs. You can also dedicate a section in your existing journal for this exercise.

STRESS JOURNAL **

Day: _____

Describe a stressful event:

_____

_____

Describe how you responded to the event:

_____

_____

How could you have avoided the situation?

_____

_____

Is this stressor something that you can avoid in the future?

_____

If yes, how? _____

_____

How can your family or loved one help you minimize this stress?

_____

_____

Did you experience any symptoms as a result of this stressful situation? _____ If yes, what were your symptoms?

_____

_____

Just like the "Symptom Log," you can make a copy of this form and use it every day for 60 days. You may want to designate a specific time each week to discuss your "Stress Log" with your family. Putting this "appointment" on your calendar will increase the likelihood of the meeting occurring. Going over your "Stress Log" with your family will allow them to better understand your experiences and help you to come up with ways that will make you feel supported in reducing the stressful events in your life.

The Prescription Option

If you're feeling overcome by anxiety, it can be extremely difficult to calm down and focus enough to benefit from a stress management routine. Up to this point, all of the stress reduction suggestions have been techniques that you can incorporate into your life and learn on your own, but sometimes the extra help of anti-anxiety medication is needed. Medication can regulate your adrenaline and help you feel a more immediate sense of control. You should consult your physician if you feel that stress is affecting your ability to function.

Responding Versus Reacting

This chapter has provided you with ways to *respond* to life and its stressors. There is a difference between *responding* to and *reacting* to life. When you *respond* to situations, you're thoughtful and deliberate. When you *react*, you go on automatic pilot and you're controlled by the situation. Can you recall a time when you were almost sideswiped by a driver talking on their cell phone? If you reacted to the situation, you may have honked your horn or even made an obscene gesture out your window.

To respond in a more conscious way to the same event, it is important to notice your heart rate was increasing and to begin to take deep breaths. Then you can recognize and acknowledge that you just felt as if your life had been threatened and that this scared you witless. Your heart rate will come down quickly and you won't create additional stress by engaging in dangerous behavior or road rage. When you respond to stressful events, the experience is managed better, your stress level comes down faster, and you feel more in control.

Using these stress-management techniques allows you to *respond* to any situation, rather than *reacting* to it. This in turn, can improve both your health and emotional well-being.

chapter
seven

Identity Crisis:
Building Self-Esteem

Somehow MS has swallowed me up. I feel like a
ghost of myself.

— *Beth; age 29, nutritionist, MS patient for 3 years*

The instant we learn that we have MS, our identities are permanently altered and we begin to battle emotional demons. Our self-esteem can falter, along with our physical capacities, and we may be further injured by the humiliating reactions others have to our frailties. While we once may have felt invincible, we may now begin to feel dependent and vulnerable. As the disease impacts our lives in various ways, we're knocked off center. It's natural to ask, "Who am I now?"

You may have heard the statement, "You are not your MS." These words are meant to provide encouragement, but they can ring false. The truth is that MS can seriously erode one's sense of self. It forces us to question—sometimes daily, sometimes hourly—who we are and what we're capable of; the answer often varies.

It's difficult to maintain a strong sense of identity when your physical and mental faculties aren't cooperating. There have been many times during the course of my disease when my self-esteem

107

wavered. I've gained weight from steroid treatments that made me feel old beyond my years. During times of extreme fatigue, I've felt I had nothing of value to offer others. I was forced to leave my demanding job as a home health social worker because I was no longer able to keep up with the physical requirements. At the age of 35, I felt that my career was over. Thankfully, all these feelings eventually passed. Yet, while I was consumed in those moments, I thought they would never pass away.

Changing Our Expectations

If you've been a physically strong, independent, competitive person, having MS may make it difficult to maintain those attributes. If you've always been able to multi-task and think quickly on your feet, slowed cognitive processing may cause you to doubt yourself as you search for words that have vanished in mid-sentence.

Depending on how seriously our mobility, energy, or cognition becomes impaired, significant changes can occur in how we spend our time and conduct our relationships. Tina, a 42-year-old woman with MS, explains, "I don't know who I am anymore. I used to play soccer competitively. I was very athletic, and that's what always made me feel good about myself. While growing up, I got constant recognition for playing sports. Now just making it through the day without using my scooter is a major accomplishment. I look in the mirror and I'm out of shape. That's not me! Who is this wimp I've become?"

Tina had previously found her sense of self-worth primarily through her athletic accomplishments. As MS made it impossible for her to compete or stay in shape physically, it was a crushing blow to her ego. As long she continued to compare herself to how she used to be and to compare the body she used to have to the one she had now, Tina continued to undermine her self-esteem. It was only after she began to recognize that her brain and body were being unfairly compared to a person without MS that she was able to readjust her expectations. With support, encouragement, and practice, Tina was able to give herself the same credit for making it through a day without using a scooter as she once did for winning a killer soccer match.

As we explored the issue further, I asked Tina, "If your best friend had MS and she were struggling to make it through the day, drawing every ounce of energy just to get to the kitchen and prepare a meal without having to sit down, would you tell her she is a worthless wimp?" Tina was shocked. "Of course not," she answered, "that would be wretched." "Why, then," I asked, "would you give yourself the same message?" I suggested that Tina try not to say anything to herself that she wouldn't say to a dear loved one. This helped her to shift her perspective, and she began to treat herself with more kindness.

Self-Esteem Is an Inside Job

Many people don't realize that our self-esteem and our self-concept don't originate from our external accomplishments, but rather from the internal dialogue that we have with ourselves. Self-esteem is defined as "having a good opinion of oneself." We're responsible for forming our own opinions of ourselves for better or worse.

In *Self-Esteem*, Dr. Matthew McKay and Patrick Fanning write:

> One of the main factors differentiating humans from other animals is the awareness of self: the ability to form an identity and then attach a value to it. In other words, you have the capacity to define who you are and then decide if you like that identity or not. The problem of self-esteem is this human capacity for judgment. When you reject parts of yourself, you greatly damage the psychological structures that literally keep you alive.

Tending to our self-esteem is a big responsibility, but it is empowering to accept the realization that we get to *choose* our self-image. This means that regardless of what our abilities are or how they change, we can consciously decide to adjust our expectations of ourselves and, in turn, adjust what we value about ourselves. Unfortunately, most of us don't understand that we have this choice. Too often we stumble into an unconscious habit of beating ourselves up and expecting far too much of ourselves. We become our own worst enemy instead of our own best friend. Our "human capacity for judgment" robs us of our spirit and zest for life far more frequently than does disease.

Sammy is a 50-year-old participant in an MS support group, and he is struggling to find self-worth as his disease progresses: "I defined myself by my job and my ability to provide for my family. I believed that this was my purpose in life. But now, I'm no longer able to work. During the quiet times when I'm home alone, I begin to wonder, what is the point of me being here at all?" To his surprise, Sammy got a tremendous response from the regular attendees at the group. Each person expressed how Sammy's presence at the group each week helped them get through their own tough times. As tears welled in his eyes, Sammy began to see how he was contributing to his community.

Do you criticize yourself because MS has diminished your abilities? Do you hear a nagging voice that says you just aren't as smart, as fast, or as useful as you used to be? This practice of "self-rejecting" is emotionally destructive and doesn't support your health in any way. To determine if you may be sending yourself critical messages, ask:

"How, specifically, has MS changed the way I see myself?"

_____

"What are some of the undermining messages I send to myself?"

_____

_____

_____

It might be helpful to share your responses with a loved one, in order to gain insight into how your limitations are perceived by *others*. You may be surprised to learn that your family and friends don't notice the differences that you perceive or they may view the changes in a more positive light than you're able to see at this time. Sharing your thoughts about how you see yourself now can be the first step you take toward rebuilding your sense of self.

Silencing Your Inner Critic

If you find that you're sending yourself negative messages, defending yourself against negative self-talk will be necessary in order to maintain a healthy sense of self. You will need to take intentional, proactive steps to silence your inner critic. In their book *Self-Esteem*, Drs. Matthew McKay and Patrick Fanning suggest that the next time you hear negative messages whispering in your ear, try the following:

- ❖ Close your eyes and take some deep breaths. Draw the air deep into your abdomen so that your diaphragm can stretch and relax.

- ❖ Relax your body. Notice and eliminate any tension in your legs and arms, your face, jaw, neck, and shoulders.

- ❖ Notice where you feel depression or criticism in your body. For instance, many people will get a stomachache or headache when they are down or feeling criticized. Sometimes this can feel like a heaviness in the limbs or even pain in the back. Focus on that place and really get to know the feeling there.

- ❖ Listen to the thoughts that go with the feeling in that part of your body. Notice everything that you're saying to yourself. Next, try to remember how the feeling began and what the self-critic was saying then.

By becoming aware of your negative self-talk, you can begin to fight back. Positive affirmations and thoughts are a powerful way to do this. The following are affirmations you can use to block out the inner-critic's voice. You may want to write these affirmations on a sticky-note and post them up on your bathroom mirror to be reminded of them daily.

The value of my life is simply that I exist.

I'm worthwhile because I am a human being.

I feel pain, love, and a range of human emotions, and at my core, I'm a good person.

I'm connected to every other person in the web of life.

I am doing the very best I can in this moment.

Everything will be O.K.

It is important that these positive affirmations mean something to you. Ask yourself what you need to hear to feel better. What would you like someone to say to you when you're down? What would you tell a friend who was not feeling good about themselves? Try to fill in the following blank:

"When I'm down, I wish someone would just tell me:

"_____."

This can become your personal affirmation that you can use anytime you're feeling insecure. Another self-healing exercise might be to offer yourself forgiveness. For example, you might want to say: "I forgive myself for feeling tired today" or "I forgive my bladder for being weak." Treating yourself with loving kindness is an effective shield that can help protect you from self-criticism.

Part of building self-esteem requires that we make room for our authentic self to emerge, that we not be intimidated by our own potential. Unfortunately, many of us have lost our true selves over the course of our lives. We take on professional roles and family roles; we adopt a certain image and present that to society in order to gain acceptance. We begin to value ourselves based on what society tells us is valuable, not on what *we* value. We change ourselves in order to be loved or admired. This often means we place a great deal of emphasis on external appearances and achievements. As we begin to ignore essential parts of ourselves, we become disconnected from our core identity.

If this has been your pattern, having a chronic disease can shatter the illusion of who you thought you were. If you've built your self-image upon externals, you're much more susceptible to experiencing an identity crisis when you become ill. But this new vulnerability can actually help lead you back to whom you once were. It can draw you into your center, where you may find many sources of healing.

Having a serious illness like MS forces you to slow down and look inward. It demands that you re-evaluate who you've become and how you're spending your time. You may ask: What gives my life meaning? How should I spend my energy? What is my purpose in life? What are the gifts that I can share despite my disabilities? These are valuable questions to consider, but most of us are too distracted with our responsibilities and busyness to ponder the bigger questions in life. Being struck with MS can shake us up in this regard. It can lead us to a more contemplative life that awakens valuable parts of ourselves that we've allowed to fall asleep. Many actually observe that they become more alive after they're diagnosed.

For example, Cynthia, a 39-year-old MS patient and mother of two, recalls:

> I was just pushing though life, just getting through the days. Taking care of my two kids and my part-time job with the paper ate up my afternoons. I was like a hamster on a wheel, just spinning, but not really getting anywhere. MS put a halt to that spinning wheel. Suddenly, I had to give up my job. I was spending hours at home alone resting. I was thinking seriously about things for the first time in years. I realized that no one was winning in this game I was playing. My kids were being cheated, my husband was being cheated, and I was being cheated. I would just rush my boys out the door in the morning, after slapping cereal on the table; my mind was always on the next thing I had to do, the next deadline. All the precious moments were just slipping by.
>
> MS made me really think about what I was missing and about what I might miss in the future. I wanted to be there as much as I could for my family. I wanted them to feel my pres-

ence and I wanted to feel theirs. I realized that taking the time to actually look into my kids' eyes when I spoke to them and listen to what they said was the greatest gift I could give them. I wasn't doing that. The extra money that I made from my job couldn't buy what my kids were missing from me. I don't know if I would've seen this about my life if MS hadn't walked in and made me slow down.

How have you been defining yourself: breadwinner, competent money manager, super-mom, hard worker, fabulous entertainer, exercise fanatic? Where have you been getting your self-worth? Is it external or internal? Through the crisis of MS, it is possible to recreate who you are in a positive and healthy way by shifting your focus from external achievements toward internal successes.

Like Cynthia, it is not uncommon for people to say that MS gives them a greater appreciation for the little things in life. This might mean that you slow down long enough to enjoy a piece of music or watch the changes that your garden goes through each season. Some say they become better listeners, more in touch with those around them and with the needs of others. As Cynthia described earlier, she took the time to look her children in the eyes when they spoke. Another woman in her early twenties explains, "MS gave me increased clarity about what is real and important in my life. I had forgotten how to enjoy the little things, like taking time to have a cup of coffee with a friend. It gave me permission to start taking care of myself again and to find joy in the simplest things. I feel older, but I also feel wiser because of this disease."

Others recognize that living with their illness makes them more compassionate and empathetic toward the suffering of others. These are just some of the valuable lessons that living with a chronic illness can teach us once we loosen our grip on our previous definitions of ourselves.

In an effort to reconnect with inherent parts of yourself that may have become dormant, I suggest you try this next exercise. Take a moment to complete an inventory of your gifts and talents. Give some thought to how you might contribute to the world in new and manageable ways. You may want to recall some special skill you had when you were younger, a hobby you enjoyed, or a talent that got neglected once you grew up and became too busy for small pleasures. I've had clients take up beading, flower arranging, photography, writing, scrap-booking, acting, gardening, cooking, painting, pottery—it really doesn't matter what you do, as long as it is something that makes you feel good about yourself when you do it. If you have trouble getting started, call a childhood friend or parent or sibling and ask them about your talents or interests during your early years. You may uncover some long-lost passions.

TALENTS AND GIFTS INVENTORY **

When I was young, my favorite way to spend time was:

Growing up, people often thought I would become a:

Some of the things I wish I had more time for are:

If I could take a class in any subject, it would be:

I've always been good at:

The one activity that absorbs me so totally I lose track of time is:

I feel good about myself when I am:

Others appreciate me for:

My life would be richer if I could:

_____

_____

_____

As you review your answers, what have you learned about yourself? Do you see a recurring interest emerging? If so, commit to taking one specific step toward adding that activity to your life. Make space for small pleasures. You will feel better about who you are when you engage in something that you love. If you believe your MS symptoms would prevent you from pursuing an activity, be proactive. Go see an occupational therapist. Ask for whatever help you might need to allow you to pursue this passion. I've been deeply inspired by the creative ideas people come up with in order to squeeze joy out of their lives. They build raised beds to help them garden, act in community theatre while in wheelchairs, or remodel their homes so they can pursue cooking. Identifying and pursuing a passion, no matter what the barrier, is a powerful boost to self-esteem.

Give of Yourself

Another way to feel better about yourself is to give of yourself. When you're feeling like you have nothing to offer because you're no longer physically able to hold down a job, or do the social scene, it may be time to explore volunteering.

Not only does volunteering increase your self-esteem, it has been proven to improve your health. Volunteering can generate a heightened sense of self-worth and confidence, reduce heart rate and blood pressure, and increase endorphin production—resulting in greater feelings of well-being and calm. Giving of your time can also boost the function of your immune system and nervous system. In addition, it can reduce stress and overcome social isolation, according to studies done by the Ontario Association of Volunteer Centers.

Psychology Today reports that researchers have actually coined the term "Helper's High" to describe how volunteers benefit from assisting others. Volunteers frequently say that they come away from the experience feeling physically, emotionally, and intellectually recharged. It seems that volunteering can meet many needs for all those involved.

I'm amazed by how my clients contribute their talents to the world. Alexis, a former elementary-school teacher, eventually developed cognitive impairments that were devastating for her. She had been a woman who thrived on intellectual stimulation, and she took great pride in her intellect. When she had to give up her teaching job, she sank into deep despair. Her self-esteem suffered greatly because she was no longer able to hold her own with the sixth-graders.

Alexis had knitted all her life. She could go through the repetitive motions of knitting without much thought. This practice gave her great comfort and peace when she felt distressed. She also felt productive and gained a sense of accomplishment when knitting. One day while having lunch with a former colleague, Alexis suggested on a whim that she come back to the elementary school to teach knitting to hyperactive kids who had trouble sitting still in class. After some brainstorming and working out of the logistics, Alexis found herself back in the classroom as a volunteer. As it turned out, the knitting had a meditative effect on the kids as well, and she developed a highly sought after program that was incorporated into many schools.

Other MS patients who are homebound have become peer counselors for their local MS society. They talk with newly diagnosed patients over the phone and share their experience, strength, and hope. Offering their unique perspective and understanding gives reassurance and validation to other MS patients, and it makes the volunteers feel valued and appreciated. It's a win-win situation for both sides.

There are numerous ways to get involved and help others. Author Jackie Waldman, who also has MS, profiles many of the ways MS patients can contribute to others in her book *People with MS with the Courage to Give.* Despite their illness, the people who tell their stories in this book managed to find creative and inspirational ways to give back to their communities. These stories are proof that no matter how MS changes your life, you can still find ways to help improve the lives of others. You may find the motivation you need to get started by reading Jackie's book.

Naturally, you will want to match your interest and skills with the particular organization you offer to help. If you love to read, see if the library needs assistance. If you used to play a sport, explore coaching. If animals give you comfort, talk with the humane society. When you reach out to help someone else, you will gain as much or more than you give from the experience.

You Are the Company You Keep

On days when your self-esteem is low, it is important to surround yourself with upbeat people whom you find encouraging and supportive. We absorb that which is reflected by others. If you're around negative people, or worse yet, people who are critical and judgmental of you, it is time to seriously re-think those relationships. It's typically better to be alone than to be with someone who brings you down and makes you feel badly about yourself.

In this chapter you've learned several techniques to combat low self-esteem. As you begin to recognize your self-worth and to feel better about yourself, it will become easier to cope with life's challenges.

Good Grief:
Recognizing the Grieving Process

Each time I feel like I've finished grieving,
MS takes something else away.
Does it ever stop?

— *Sally; age 39, elementary school teacher,*
MS patient for 7 years

The diagnosis of a chronic illness completely disrupts our life. The future we envisioned may suddenly be altered. Getting sick was not part of our plan! The loss of our healthy self requires that we reconstruct our internal world: a struggle we re-encounter with each downturn in our illness. And we do it. As human beings, we instinctively strive to regain our balance. We search for ways to assimilate painful situations into our lives, and we're compelled to begin the process of integrating traumatic events into our psyche.

Even when we experience losses of great magnitude, we eventually recognize that we must go on, find new meaning in our lives, and feel productive. Eventually, your attitude toward your altered life can be successfully transformed, but first you must go through the grieving process.

Grief Is a Response to Any Loss

The loss of a loved one is not the only situation that can cause sorrow or grief. Grieving is a normal response to *any* significant loss. While coping with MS, the grieving process is a tool that allows us to revise our view of ourselves and reorganize our life in order to adapt to our losses. We were designed to grieve, just as we were designed to laugh and love.

Grief allows us to survive change and MS patients have many opportunities to become skilled in its use. The protracted course and chronic nature of this illness require that we grieve many times, for many losses. Few other illnesses cause more ongoing feelings of loss than MS. Every new symptom represents a loss that must be acknowledged and absorbed.

When we recognize the need to grieve and give ourselves permission to acknowledge our losses, we're able to move beyond overwhelming feelings of helplessness toward a feeling of control and a healthy perspective. Sometimes, however, it can be difficult to identify or articulate what we've lost. This can be especially true for cognitive and sexual losses. These are sensitive subjects that can be very difficult to deal with. Since they can be awkward to talk about (and therefore to get support for), often these losses leave people feeling even more isolated in their grief.

COGNITIVE LOSSES

Holly, a single woman in her late twenties with MS, mourns every time her disease takes a turn for the worse:

> Most people think that the hardest part of having MS has been my need for a walker, but I coped with that. Walking became more difficult over several years and I had time to adjust to it. It's what they don't see that eats me up. I just can't think or reason the way I used to. It feels as if I've lost my spark and personality. The quick, witty comments that were my trademark humor now elude me. I feel like a bump on a log when I get together with friends. I can't remember the last conversation we had or what's going on in their lives. It isn't that I don't care. I just can't remember. How do you explain this to people?

For many patients like Holly, cognitive losses are more difficult to accept than the more apparent physical limitations. We define our sense of self by our ability to think, to reason, and to communicate with others, and when this ability is compromised, it can feel as if a critical part of who we are has disappeared. This is a very real loss that is often difficult for others to understand.

SEXUAL LOSSES

Steven, a 49-year-old man with MS, confesses, "If I had to name one thing that has been the most difficult to let go of, it would be my manhood. Not only has MS interfered with my ability to provide financially for my family, but I've experienced sexual dysfunction as well. My wife is wonderful about it, but that has been a huge blow to my ego—a big loss."

The loss of our sexual selves is a frequent problem for MS patients and it can have complicated consequences. However, this is another loss that patients find embarrassing and difficult to discuss. We will address this significant issue in further detail in Chapter 11.

Sometimes, when we feel alone in our losses, it can help to remember that loss is a universal experience. We begin life with the loss of the warm, nourishing womb and end life with the loss of all we have come to know and love. Mourning our losses is an essential task for growth and maturity. It's a fact of life for all of us.

The Stages of Grief

What do we know about grief? Over the years, a general consensus has emerged that suggests we go through predictable stages of mourning. Psychiatrist Elisabeth Kübler-Ross wrote the highly acclaimed *On Death and Dying*, which greatly influenced our understanding of the grieving process. Kübler-Ross suggests that we experience five specific stages of grief, and although her work focused on death, these five stages are now commonly recognized as being present during any loss.

DENIAL

Denial is the first stage. For many MS patients denial may occur when they are first diagnosed. Initially we think, "There must be some mistake." Or, during the course of our illness, we may ignore the fact that we have the disease until it gets our attention during an exacerbation. Denial can be an effective coping mechanism, allowing our psyche time to catch up with reality.

ANGER

Anger (at doctors, God, ourselves) comes next. Inevitably we ask, "Why me?" We may lash out at those who try to comfort or support us and alienate those we love. At times, anger can be blinding and prevent us from seeing light at the end of the tunnel, but it can also be necessary to give us strength and power when we need it the most.

BARGAINING

Bargaining is the third response. When we try to cut deals with fate, we are attempting to avoid the inevitable: "If you just get me through this episode, I swear I'll change my lifestyle and stop pushing myself so hard." Once we recover from a relapse, we often tempt fate again and renege on our bargain, going back to our old unhealthy ways and habits.

DEPRESSION OR SADNESS

The fourth stage, depression, occurs when we really feel current and past losses, and perhaps anticipate new ones. I would describe this stage as sadness, rather than depression, because eventually you do move through this stage, and it is a necessary, healthy part of the grieving process. This is the time when we need to feel our sadness and just *be* with it.

ACCEPTANCE

The final stage is acceptance. However, Kübler-Ross cautions that "This stage should not be mistaken for a happy phase." This is a time that seems almost void of emotion. The struggle is over and we accept our situation. Once we reach this stage, we may finally be able to move forward and no longer feel consumed with grief.

Although experts agree that most of us do experience these feelings while mourning, critics say that these stages are not predictable. I concur. Just like MS, the process may not be linear. We may bounce from one stage to another or regress from acceptance to denial. This is particularly true for those who must grieve many losses.

The Symptoms of Grief

Feelings that may emerge when grieving include apathy, anxiety, irritability, longing, vulnerability, dependency, a sense of meaninglessness, shock, humiliation, and avoidance. Obviously, a wide range of emotions accompanies grief.

Furthermore, don't be surprised to experience physical symptoms as you grieve. The body reacts to intense feelings of mourning. It is not unusual to cry and sigh or to feel tightness in the throat, shortness of breath, restlessness, aches and pains, sleeplessness, and extreme fatigue. Writer Joan Didion aptly describes grief in her book *The Year of Magical Thinking:* "Grief comes in waves, paroxysms, sudden apprehensions that weaken the knees, and blind the eyes and obliterate the dailiness of life."

You may not be prepared for the intensity or duration of your emotions, or for how swiftly your feelings change. Some people can even begin to doubt their sanity when going through intense grief. Although grief can make you feel like you are going crazy, this is a natural process. Please be assured that these feelings are healthy and even necessary in order for you to come to terms with your losses.

If we aren't allowed to fully experience our grief, we may suffer from complicated grief, which keeps us mired in bitterness or sadness. Complicated grief is a grief that's compounded and stifled by conflicting feelings or denial. When our grief is complicated, it can be stalled and prevent us from moving through the process toward healing. As with the other emotions we experience, what's important is that the loss be acknowledged by ourselves and, if possible, others. This recognition helps us to move through the grief process.

When We Grieve

For many, the initial diagnosis of MS is their first significant loss. This is the time when you grapple with the fact that you're the same person, yet you're different. Your previous image of yourself must be adjusted to make room for the effect MS will have on you. Once this task is accomplished, you're released to go on with your life while making any changes that are necessary to accommodate your illness.

It's also common for grief to occur during exacerbations. This is when we're forced to cope with the unique challenges of MS. Perhaps we began to feel that we had the disease under control or that we were misdiagnosed. Some people come to believe that if they follow certain "rules," such as eliminating stress, taking their medication, and following a healthy diet, they will avoid having further attacks. And in some cases this is true for a while. So when you've been in remission for a period of time and then a new flare-up forces you to face the fact that you're truly living with an incurable chronic illness, it can feel like a sucker punch to the gut. Once more, we may find ourselves grieving all over again. Depending on the length of time between exacerbations, we may no sooner have accepted one consequence before our illness imposes yet another hurdle. This can be an unbelievably frustrating experience.

If we're left with some residual disability after an exacerbation, such as an impairment of eyesight or mobility, we may need to grieve the loss of that particular physical ability. Each one of these new symptoms brings with it ramifications that can affect your life in many ways. You may have to give up driving, or reading, or working. These are very real losses that must be grieved as they arise.

Melinda, an MS patient in her sixties, explains, "It seems that each time I have another attack, I'm thrown off guard. Just when I think I have this thing under control, it pulls on my shirtsleeve to remind me it is still there. Every time something else goes wrong, I feel like a chair has been knocked out from under me."

Physical changes aren't the only losses we must mourn. Some relationships become strained beyond repair. We may lose our financial security. Our independence may be compromised; our hopes for a family or dreams of a certain type of career can be shattered. It takes a great deal of strength and courage to endure all these losses, but what choice do we have?

If we're to salvage what we can from our life and continue to get the most out of what we *have* been given, we must grieve our losses, consider what we're still able to do, and move forward.

Fortunately, there are several ways to make the grieving process easier. A wonderful website, www.griefwatch.com, recommends the tips listed below. Review this list of suggestions and choose five or six that you can incorporate into your own emotional process:

GRIEVING STRATEGIES **

Admit that you're hurting and let the pain come.

Ask for and accept support.

Face the loss.

Stop asking "Why?" and instead ask, "What will I do now?"

Keep a routine even if you must force yourself to do it.

Take care of something alive, like a pet or a plant.

Apply a cold or heat pad to your body, whichever feels best.

Rest.

Know that you will survive.

Find someone who needs your help.

Don't overdo things.

Eat regularly.

Be around people.

Exercise.

Postpone making any major decisions until you feel better.

Most importantly, recognize that grief has no allotted time period. Try not to compare yourself to others. Some grieve quickly, some slowly. Allow yourself to go through the process at your own pace.

For some, grief can be compounded. If you haven't let yourself fully experience a previous loss, you could be susceptible to a snowball effect when you do finally begin to grieve. For instance, you may find yourself mourning the loss of your grandmother at the same time you're forced to give up your walking routine. Although this can seem unfair at the time, its nature's way of allowing us to release built-up sadness.

Releasing the Shame

Let me tell you a dirty little secret. For many of us, grieving involves acknowledging shameful emotions that we would rather deny. These are the ugly thoughts that sometimes accompany our feelings of loss. We may go through a period of resenting those who are caring for us, or feeling jealous toward those who still possess good health. Perhaps we dare not confess these feelings, and yet concealing them chokes us with pain and anger. You may not realize it, but these are common feelings shared by most people who suffer from a chronic illness.

Being vulnerable makes you mad. Kathy, a 48-year-old MS patient, explains:

> Initially, all I could feel was rage toward my disease, my doctor, and even my husband who patiently gave me care and support. Each time I had to ask for help or suffered another attack, I would become furious. Each step back seemed like a direct affront to my dignity and I would lash out at those who loved me the most. Then, during the course of one year, I had two friends

die of breast cancer and one friend lose her husband to an aneurysm. This was my wake-up call. I realized that I had a right to my anger and sadness, but if I wanted to overcome my rage, I needed to feel grateful for what I *did* have. It all changed for me that year. I made a conscious decision to take delight in the abilities I still had. I took up writing and went to some classes at the community college. I even got my husband to join me since he had to drive me there anyway. It seems like gratitude was what released me from my grief. It's been a good trade.

Eventually, Kathy became a master at accommodating the successive losses exacted by her MS, but first it took witnessing the losses of others for her to begin her own healing. We're not saints. We will all have these negative feelings at some point. The goal is to acknowledge them, release them, and let them pass so that you can once again participate in the joy of living and loving.

Attitude of Gratitude

As we look for ways to move beyond our grief, the theme of gratitude often makes an appearance. Discovering the grace of gratitude when facing the many losses imposed by chronic illness can be a miraculous way of compensating. Shifting one's attention from what you've lost toward what you still have is a significant step toward achieving the final stage of grief: acceptance. Our ability to live a fulfilling life despite our disease will arise directly from our appreciation of each function we're able to retain and by recognizing the new skills we acquire.

The next time you find yourself facing another loss or feeling hopeless, it might help to compile a gratitude list. Simply take a moment at the beginning of your day to make a list of all the things for which you are grateful. One example might look like this:

**GRATITUDE LIST **

The sun is out.

My cat is with me in bed.

I have food in the refrigerator.

My house is warm.

I have a phone, and I can call someone if I desire.

My best friend is coming over for tea.

My pain is only at a level three today.

I have a good book to read.

I have an invitation to spend Christmas with someone I care about.

I didn't wake up with a cold.

This gives you some idea of the simple gifts we are given every day. Even the smallest pleasures can be appreciated when we take a moment to be aware of what we have. Sometimes, we must slow down so that we are able to see the many gifts we are given each day. Try to write out a gratitude list each morning for the next week and see how you feel afterward.

If you find yourself feeling critical or negative during the day, shift your attention to something for which you're grateful. See if your body does not become more relaxed and your breathing more steady. Be attuned to how your feelings shift when you focus on the gifts in your life. This is living consciously. The simple act of paying attention to your thoughts and feelings and choosing to be grateful can re-direct your emotions toward a healthy course.

Another way to acknowledge gratitude is to give some type of blessing before each meal. Express your gratitude for the nourishment you are about to receive. This doesn't necessarily need to be a religious blessing (although it could be), but simply a statement of appreciation for the food on your table. For instance, some cultures like to recognize the animal or plant life that was given for the sustenance we receive at each meal. This symbolic gesture helps to bring us out of ourselves and encourages us to feel a connection with the rest of the world or with a power greater than ourselves. Saying a blessing helps us to feel cared for and provided for even when it seems that so much has been taken away.

The Importance of Ritual

Rituals ground us during periods of grief. Almost every culture in the world calls for a form of ritual to be performed when someone dies. These rituals provide a way to contain sadness, and they offer a purpose and direction for the bereaved.

After living in the South for many years and attending a few memorial services, I was struck by the Southern ritual of preparing and providing food for family members who had lost a loved one. At first, I thought that all these people constantly dropping by with impossible amounts of pie and casserole might be an imposition. The grief-stricken wife or husband was required to receive these visitors and then figure out what the heck to do with all the food for which they had no appetite. Not to mention that they had to get all the dishes back to the rightful owners. Yet it soon became clear to me that these gestures not only made the bereaved feel loved and cared for, it also gave them something to do. It forced mourners to write thank-you notes and to stay involved with the community. These basic rules of etiquette connected the bereaved to reality when everything else seemed unreal.

Rituals can serve the same purposes when grieving over MS losses. The road to resilience begins with keeping a routine and committing to something that has always been familiar. You may want to pick one or two things that remain constant while you're grieving. This might include walking your dog twice a day or having a cup of tea and listening to classical music at 4:00 P.M. every afternoon, or writing in your journal. For some, religious practices can bring great comfort. The symbolic act of lighting a candle and taking a moment to get centered can provide steady reassurance when everything else feels off-kilter. Whatever your habits have been over the years, you must hang on to them during the times of grief when so many other things seem to be changing.

Patty, a 33-year-old with chronic-progressive MS, explains, "Ever since I was a child I've written poetry. This was my escape and my comfort, especially when tension got thick between my parents. Writing has been my one constant thread throughout life.

I've lost a great deal, but now that I'm confined to my home, I have all the time I've always wanted to do what I love—write."

Gaining Through Loss

Patty's story is a good example of how during our losses we may benefit in ways we had never considered before. A tipping point is often reached during the mourning process. Suddenly, you may find yourself laughing again or taking an interest in activities and friends. Gradually, we re-emerge from our despair, and although some aspects of ourselves are changed forever, we may also discover positive ways to live in our new circumstances.

On many occasions, clients have told me that having a chronic illness is actually a gift. This shift in perception rarely comes from passive endurance. A decisive choice is made to explore what can be done to make the best out of a bad situation. This may be a very difficult concept to warm up to, but give it a chance. If we are to endure the complexities of this illness, we must be flexible enough to open ourselves up to new possibilities.

I've personally experienced how MS can be a motivator to move dreams or ambitions forward. The first year I was diagnosed, my husband and I began to talk about what was truly important to us. Knowing that we could no longer take my health for granted, we set some goals. We shared a dream of taking a year off to travel. Suddenly, it became clear to us that we shouldn't wait to make this happen. Who knows how healthy either of us would be by the time we reached retirement? Once we got the notion, we took the steps to make it happen. We rented out our house and car, found a very dear friend to take care of our dog PK, and my husband's company agreed to pay for our health insurance as long as he was willing to return to his job when the year was up. We were going to live our dream.

The trip was the most spectacular experience of our lives. We visited 17 different countries and met incredible people from diverse cultures. Living out of our backpacks and staying in hostels, we learned how little we really needed to be happy.

Nothing can take away the memories we created during that trip. After planning and executing our adventure, I developed greater confidence. I realized that when I set my mind on doing something, I could do it. I don't know if we ever would have made that dream a reality if I hadn't gotten MS.

Humans have a natural tendency to avoid facing the reality that all of us will one day be physically limited by age or disease. Chronic illness challenges this complacency and can bring to life desires that we had let go dormant.

When illness upsets the rhythm of our lives, we can use the situation to our advantage. For 22 years, Ellen worked as an accountant. She sat at a computer every day without any windows to bring in daylight. After living with MS for several years, she eventually began to have cognitive problems that interfered with her ability to work with numbers. Initially, she was fearful. "How will we make ends meet? I'm not ready to retire," she cried as she sat in my office. Ellen had to grieve the loss of her life as she knew it before she was ready to consider new possibilities for herself. In time, she was able to begin exploring other options for employment. Ellen had always dreamed of working in a nursery. Her inspiration came from a beautiful garden store that was just a few blocks from her home. She would often stop by there after work and pick out a few gorgeous blooming plants to add some color to her drab and lifeless cubical. After some encouragement, she asked if the store needed any help and before she knew what happened, she was working there two days a week.

Her interactions with people and caring for the plants brought Ellen more joy than she had ever experienced in her previous job where she worked amid balance sheets and stressed out coworkers. A few months later, her daughter asked if she'd be willing to babysit two days a week. Ellen was thrilled to spend more one-on-one time with her precious granddaughter. MS forced Ellen to make changes that enhanced her life in ways she would have been unable to imagine when she was mourning the loss of her job.

On a less dramatic scale, the writer May Sarton speaks of appreciating the smallest things while suffering from an illness: "I panted halfway up the stairs, but I also was able to sit and watch light change on the porch for over an hour and be truly attentive to it, not plagued by what I 'ought' to be doing." Ms. Sarton had lost her ability to easily ascend the stairs, but she found her powers of observation enhanced by releasing herself from the mundane demands of life. Her illness gave her an excuse to ignore the "oughts."

This isn't to suggest that having a chronic disease makes everyone's life better. It makes it different and painful and difficult, but once we beat our chests and shed our tears over what we've lost, we must begin to actively search out what we might gain.

How *You* Grieve

In this section you're encouraged to identify your own way of grieving. Some of the guidelines given in this chapter can help you recognize signs and patterns of grief; however, you may have developed your own unique way of mourning loss over the course of your lifetime. Take a moment to explore the following questions about how you grieve. You can write the answers in your journal.

GRIEF QUESTIONNAIRE **

Describe the first loss you ever experienced.

How did you express your feelings at the time?

What happened in your family when someone died?

How did your family teach you to grieve?

How were you comforted during your first loss?

How do you comfort others when they grieve?

What do you need most when you're grieving?

Do you agree with Dr. Kübler-Ross's stages of grief?

If not, how is the process different for you?

How do you know when you're grieving?

In what part(s) of your body do you feel grief most powerfully?

What rituals do you follow that might help you during loss?

How do you know when you're starting to heal from loss?

What has been your greatest loss so far?

What loss do you fear the most?

Answering these questions will help raise your awareness about how you grieve. Examining your past experiences can teach you about your own beliefs and enable you to better recognize when you've suffered a loss. Once we acknowledge that we've suffered a loss, it becomes easier to give ourselves the space and time needed to mourn.

Moving Forward

After we've permitted ourselves to mourn, the time will come for us to let go and embrace life, despite what we've lost. In *Kitchen Table Wisdom*, Dr. Rachel Naomi Remen warns us of the dangers that lurk when we refuse to separate from what we once had:

> Sometimes we may simply have to choose life. It's possible to become so attached to something or someone we have lost that we move forward blindly, looking over our shoulder to the past rather than before us to what lies ahead. The Bible tells us that as she looked back, Lot's wife was turned into a pillar of salt. I suspect that many of us have had this happen to us without our realizing that we have become frozen, trapped by the past. We are holding on to something long gone and, hands full, are unable to take hold of our opportunities or what life is offering.

I encourage you to see beyond what once was and discover the possibilities of what might be yet to come.

Perhaps you've never even considered this question, but could you have possibly benefited in any way from your illness? This may seem counterintuitive, but spend a moment to try and identify three things that you've gained because of your MS.

THREE GIFTS MS HAS GIVEN ME *

1. _____

2. _____

3. _____

The gifts you identify can be extraordinarily simple and yet immensely enriching.

In my case, I've found that MS helps me to more clearly identify my needs. I know what I need to do to take care of myself and feel I have the right to ask for what I require to stay healthy. I've become more vulnerable, and this has allowed me to let my friends and family get closer to me. Having MS has given me the opportunity to reach out and offer understanding to others who also have the disease. These gifts are profound and have greatly expanded my life. Yet I had to consider the question, "What has MS given me?" before I was able to clearly see the positive ways the illness had changed my life. Asking this question will open your consciousness to the possibility that some good can come out of tragedy. It often takes a willingness to explore the positive side of things for grace to appear.

Sharing these answers with your loved ones, and exploring how this exercise makes you feel, may give others a deeper understanding of what you're experiencing. It might be helpful to ask them if *they* can see any benefits from your having the disease as well. My husband remarked that he enjoys the fact that I'm home more often and less distracted and stressed by my job. He feels MS has helped me make our relationship my top priority, rather than my work. I don't know if I would've necessarily viewed it this way, but I'm glad that he does.

Life truly is about living with a sense of transience, knowing that however much we treasure a person or situation or ability, eventually things will change. And although we're powerless to stop loss from occurring, we can choose how we grieve. We can decide to feel our despair and then focus on hope.

Sick and Tired of
Feeling Sick and Tired

I can't stand it when healthy people say, "I get tired
too." My MS causes a bone-tired, hit-the-wall kind of
fatigue. They have no understanding of what it's like.
When it hits, it stops you in your tracks.

— *Amy; age 48, salesperson, MS patient for 15 years*

Although the experience of fatigue varies, it generally has an enormous impact on MS patients. Reports indicate that about 78 percent of the MS population suffers from fatigue, and patients claim of all MS symptoms, fatigue causes the greatest limitations.

It's difficult for others to understand the level of fatigue that MS patients endure. For the person who doesn't struggle with illness, fatigue is something that can be pushed through or ignored when duty calls. Not so with MS. The type of fatigue that MS imposes can't be argued with. It will land you flat on your back and knock you out cold in the middle of the day. It can make taking a shower or brushing your teeth feel like a major accomplishment. It can come on suddenly at the most inconvenient times. It makes us feel weak and grouchy. We may wake up tired after having a full night's sleep and continue to feel tired for many days to come, no matter how much we rest. Is it any wonder that we get sick and tired of feeling sick and tired?

MS Fatigue Cannot Be Underestimated

MS fatigue is often pervasive, chronic, and can last the entire course of the disease. Some patients live with a feeling of exhaustion much of the time; others get tired quickly, after minimal exertion. It is like a thief that robs us of our life force, making it one of the hardest symptoms to deal with emotionally. One MS patient explains:

> Fatigue is my major presenting symptom. What bothers me most is admitting that I don't have the energy to do everything and making hard choices between work and play. It took me a long time to get to the point where I could leave work early or take a day off because I had something personal to get done and didn't have the energy to take care of things after work. It's so hard trying to convey to others what MS fatigue feels like. I'm not just tired; I'm drained. I can wake up fatigued even after a good night's sleep. The fatigue can hit mid-sentence and I can literally feel myself drooping.

MS fatigue is hard to describe. When I've overdone it, I experience a bone-numbing tiredness that makes movement seem impossible. Because MS fatigue varies so dramatically, it can be impossible to know from day-to-day what our capabilities will be. Someone with MS can walk without assistance early in the day and require a wheelchair, or even be bedridden, by evening because of fatigue. Both planning and "going with the flow" become a necessary part of every activity. Glena, a 44-year-old patient, describes her experience with fatigue:

> I plan my days and my weeks in advance so that I spread out the important events that I want to attend and have the energy to do them. I try to take naps on days that I know will be stressful. When it comes to deciding whether to rest ahead or crash later, well sometimes I do both. There are days when you just have to give in to it and live with the fact that you can accom-

plish very little. I try to be flexible with my schedule so that it allows for rescheduling things. I do get frustrated when I try to keep up with my healthy friends and family members. Sometimes it makes me really angry.

We all try to find ways to accommodate fatigue, and that often means making compromises. Another MS patient responds, "I rest up in advance of activities and then if I'm not up to it when the time comes, I just don't do it. I just can't pay the price of the consequences when I overdo it. Fortunately, the friends I have love me, care about me, and understand."

MS fatigue is unlike any other. As you may have experienced, this type of fatigue impacts every aspect of life. Our work, family, friends, activities, and our emotional health all suffer from our feelings of exhaustion. Naturally, fatigue changes our personality. During periods of tiredness, we can become an entirely different person than we were just hours earlier. Like a small child who has missed a nap, we may become cranky, sullen, sensitive, needy, weepy, worried, or pessimistic. We tend to draw into ourselves and avoid social situations because we don't have the energy to interact with others. If we're socializing and feel tired, we may seem disinterested or distracted and be judged unfairly. We may be less likely to go the extra mile for friends and family even when we truly want to extend ourselves. Sometimes we snap at our loved ones or just retreat to the bedroom, shutting the door behind us.

Betty, a 28-year-old MS patient, tries to explain to her family how her experience of fatigue brings out the worst in her:

> The hardest part of this disease to accept is not having the energy I should at my age. I don't have the energy to do simple daily tasks, let alone reach my goals and dreams. I get so tired so fast, it's extremely frustrating. I fight my lack of energy and I push myself. I tell myself, "I'm not crippled, everyone else can do it, and I should be able to do it also." Then I get *really* tired and lose my grip and the smallest things set me off.
>
> What I need for everyone to understand is that I'm not really reacting to little things; I'm reacting to the fact that I'm exhausted and can't take anymore. When that happens, even one

more little thing becomes the last straw. Deep inside I'm reacting to the fact that I hate always being tired, that I hate dealing with the little details, and somehow this hate has to come
out. I just need for everyone to understand how hard dealing
with all this is for me.

As Betty eloquently explains, over time this cycle of exhaustion
can become demoralizing. Our confidence and our ability to keep
things in perspective may slip away. We may also be more sensitive
to innocent remarks because we're less able to control our moods
when MS fatigue sweeps in.

It stands to reason that if we're dog-tired, our motivation and
creativity are stifled. When it is all we can do to just get through
the day, exercise programs falter and projects around the house go
untouched. Bosses may think we're lazy because we're slower to accomplish tasks at work. We may need to take more breaks during
the day. Often, we end up feeling as if we're not doing anything
well. When every aspect of life is affected by our exhaustion, it is
easy to understand why fatigue is perceived as the most debilitating symptom for most MS patients.

Understanding the insidious nature of MS fatigue can help us
to be more forgiving of ourselves and to better explain to others
what our weariness feels like.

Physical vs. Mental Fatigue

Symptoms of fatigue can actually be broken down into two categories: physical fatigue and mental fatigue.

Physical fatigue is usually experienced as reduced stamina and
exhaustion that is beyond what you would normally expect from
doing an activity. There may be no correlation between the amount
of energy you exert and the extent of your lethargy. For instance,
you may start off on a short walk and feel full of energy. However,
shortly after you begin to stroll, your may find that your gait begins
to deteriorate, you feel off balance, and your legs get so heavy that
you have to take a break and rest. When you try to ignore your

physical symptoms and push on, it can feel as though you've just tried to climb an imposing mountain. As one young woman with MS describes it, "I'm 35 years old, but I feel like I'm 85. There are times when I feel really good. I will have a good day and then I'm seduced into doing a little more and a little more until suddenly I'm flat on my butt. I never seem to learn how to stop *before* I get worn out."

Mental fatigue often follows on the heels of physical fatigue. However, it can be a completely separate issue as well. Although not well understood, mental fatigue is a common experience for many MS patients. The medical community now acknowledges that MS hampers thought processes as well as movement. Just like with physical symptoms, the quality and clarity of thinking in MS patients can vary. Someone who can balance their checkbook in the early morning may space out and forget their own phone number by the end of the day.

Tasks that would not normally take much mental exertion, such as following directions or discussing the family budget, can feel beyond our ability when we're tired. Like physical fatigue, the intensity of mental fatigue is far greater than what is typically experienced by people without the disease. Patients often report that overstimulation can trigger brain fog, due to the noise in a crowded restaurant or multi-tasking, for example.

When patients pay close attention, they often find that mental fatigue follows a pattern. Many recognize that they feel energized early in the day, but by late afternoon or evening, they can barely function. Napping at a predictable hour tends to help these patients get a second wind later in the day.

Unlike cognitive impairments, mental fatigue will normally subside with rest.

In general, MS fatigue does not appear to be related to any level of disability or physical functioning. Someone may be confined to a wheelchair but not experience any fatigue, while another patient may have good physical mobility, but be unable to complete common daily tasks because of weariness.

Why Am I So Tired?

Why do you feel so tired? The answer is multi-faceted. Sometimes the demyelination and inflammation associated with MS can be the culprit. Chronic pain, weakened muscles, medication side effects, sleep disruption, and emotional issues (such as depression and anxiety) can also play a role. It's important to rule out the possibility of other diseases that may cause extreme fatigue as well.

Understanding the root cause of fatigue can help alleviate the guilt you might feel about being tired so often and validate your experience. The following six common causes of fatigue clearly explain why you're not able to just suck it up and push through your weariness.

Demyelination. The task of the brain is to send and receive signals. The spinal cord uses a network of nerves to transmit those signals to various parts of our body. The nerves are coated by a type of insulation called myelin. This protective sheath helps the nerve fibers conduct the signals throughout the body.

Problems occur when disease activity triggered by MS causes the myelin to break down and replaces it with scar tissue. This process is called demyelination, which impedes the flow of signals from the central nervous system, slowing or at times blocking vital communication. On a practical level, this can interfere with our ability to think or function.

This decrease in the brain's ability to process information is a primary cause of profound physical and mental fatigue. Your brain has to work much harder to get its messages across. Hence, you can get tired just from thinking.

As you may have experienced, this fatigue is often made worse by heat. It's believed that heat may trigger inflammation, which can further interrupt signals from the brain. Heat fatigue is typically improved by cooling off.

Deconditioning. Unfortunately, fatigue can create a vicious cycle. Until we learn to tune into our bodies and pace ourselves, we may stop doing any activity for fear of getting too tired afterwards. This decrease in activity can cause us to lose muscle strength and tone. When muscles are not worked, they tend to become weaker, creating increased fatigue and decreased stamina. As our stamina is decreases, it becomes harder to start moving again or to stay active. The best defense against deconditioning is to keep moving.

Depression. As I mentioned previously, one significant symptom of depression is fatigue. However, fatigue from depression is often not resolved with rest and does not result from over-activity or stimulation. Depression-related fatigue is normally chronic and, unlike other causes of fatigue, depression fatigue will respond to treatment with antidepressant medication and counseling.

Side Effects of Medication. If you take a look at the side effects described for most medications, drowsiness will often be listed. This is true for many of the drugs commonly used to treat MS, so it is no surprise that you may feel tired when taking certain prescriptions. If you're feeling sluggish, listen to your body and talk with your doctor. There may be strategies that you can use to minimize the impact of medication on your energy level. Ask if you're on the lowest possible effective dose. You may have to experiment with your dosage to zero-in on the best therapeutic level for you. Often, taking the medication at a different time of day can make a significant difference. If you're taking a pill before you go the bed, it may interrupt your sleep schedule, so it might be better to take it in the morning. If you're taking a pill in the morning that makes you drowsy, you may be able to take it before bedtime. Are there any alternatives to taking the medication, such as exercise, stretching, meditating, or physical therapy? It's worth exploring all these possibilities with your physician.

Pain. At least 20 to 50 percent of those with MS report significant pain. For anyone who has experienced living with chronic pain, you know it can be a terribly draining experience. It takes a considerable amount of energy to fight pain, as we try to shrink it down to a tolerable level. This leaves us with little energy to put toward anything else. Effectively using a pain management medication regime may substantially increase your energy. If you're on pain medication, it is normally recommended that you take it before your pain reaches an unbearable level. The goal is to manage the pain so that it demands less of your energy and attention.

Sleep Disruption. Sleep disorders are estimated to be three times more prevalent in MS patients than in the rest of the population. Problems with overactive bladders and frequent urination can keep patients running to the bathroom several times a night. Once you are up, it can be very difficult to go back to sleep. Muscle spasms and spasticity can also affect the quality of sleep for patients. In addition, if you get into a habit of napping later in the day or you're inactive during most of the day, it can be difficult to sleep at night. Insomnia can keep you up for hours even when you're exhausted.

One of my clients came up with the idea of keeping a bedside commode in her room at night. She found that if she didn't have to walk all the way to the bathroom, it was easier for her to get back to sleep. There are now medications such as Detrol, of the famed "Gotta go" commercials, that can be helpful in controlling bladder dysfunction. Spasticity can be controlled with the prescription Baclofen. For some, a sleep aid is appropriate. All of these medical treatments can be explored by you and your doctor.

One final suggestion: If you nap during the day, you may want experiment with napping earlier, perhaps no later than 2:00 P.M.

Addressing Fatigue

Regardless of the cause, it is important to address fatigue, because treatments and therapies can be of great benefit in managing its effects.

Unfortunately, despite the high incidence of fatigue for people with MS and having the ability to treat it, physicians often overlook or underestimate the impact of exhaustion. After telling one of my previous neurologists that I was too tired to sit up through a meal, she responded by saying that I was, after all, 43-years-old, and I should expect to feel more tired than I once did. This doctor was trying to tell me that I didn't have the stamina to make it through a meal at the dinner table because I was now in my forties! My level of fatigue was clearly not "normal" for a 43-year-old. I was tempted to ask her if she had to lie down to eat her meals since she was, after all, about my age. I share this example to illustrate how physicians may be unaware of the extent to which our lives are dramatically impacted by fatigue. I needed the neurologist to discuss ways in which we might address my fatigue, not have her minimize it and dismiss it as a normal part of aging.

Since fatigue is subjective and invisible, it is extremely difficult for physicians to fully comprehend how you may be affected by it. Once again, it will fall upon your shoulders to specifically and accurately paint a picture of how you experience fatigue.

In *Fatigue in Multiple Sclerosis*, Dr. Lauren B. Krupp lists some of the more common descriptors of fatigue. If any of these symptoms apply to you, it may be useful to tell your doctor:

❖ Physical tiredness

❖ Mental tiredness

❖ Lack of motivation

❖ Difficulty concentrating

❖ Inability to complete tasks

❖ Feelings of depression

❖ Feelings of anxiety

❖ Failure to feel refreshed after sleep

❖ Overall muscle weakness

❖ Weakness in certain muscle groups

❖ Poor performance at home or work

❖ Performance that fails to meet prior expectations

❖ Pain or physical discomfort

I would like to add a few other symptoms to this list:

❖ Feeling fuzzy-headed or foggy-brained

❖ Unable to stay awake to read or watch TV

❖ Unable to make decisions

❖ Avoiding social or work demands

❖ Sleeping or taking naps during the day

❖ Unable to exercise

❖ Exhausted by exposure to heat

Medical Treatments for Fatigue

Once your doctor recognizes the significant impact that fatigue is having on your life (and you have addressed sleep disturbances), your physician may decide to prescribe medication to help keep you alert and active during the day. Although no medication to date has been approved by the FDA to specifically treat fatigue in MS, many medicines have been prescribed over the last few decades that have proven to be helpful. There are a number of drugs you may ask your doctor about. Provigil, also knows as Modafinil, is a wake-promoting drug designed to work in areas of the brain involved in the regulation of regular wakefulness. Amantadine, an antiviral agent, is also a central nervous system stimulant, which increases dopamine levels in the brain. Dopamine facilitates communication between nerve cells. Some antidepressants have also been found to be effective, although these drugs may be most effective when depression is the underlying cause of the fatigue. As with antidepressants, you might need to experiment with the medications until you discover what works for you.

Jackie, a woman in her sixties who has had MS for years, says, "Before Provigil, I was a zombie. I couldn't take care of my grandkids, which is my greatest joy. I was just no fun to be around. After I started taking my little pep pills, life changed dramatically for me.

Travel even became possible. Sometimes I can adjust my dose depending on what I have committed to that day. This drug gave me my life back." I want to caution, however, that not everyone has this type of positive results with medication, but it is certainly worth discussing the options with your doctor.

Pacing Yourself

As with stress, it may be helpful for you to pay attention to what specifically brings on your fatigue. The degree and causes of fatigue vary for each of us, but if you know what your fatigue triggers are, you will be better able to prepare for them and pace yourself so that you don't reach the breaking point.

Assign a fatigue level to each of the following activities. A rating of one would be little or no fatigue, and 10 would be extreme fatigue. You may want to add a few extra lines for categories that are not included here. Again, you can use your journal to record your answers.

RATING YOUR FATIGUE **

Activity	Level of fatigue (1–10)
Socializing	
Exercising	
Shopping	
Traveling	
Driving	
Walking	
Making important decisions	
Working (part-time, full-time)	
Multi-tasking	
Entertaining	

(cont'd.)

RATING YOUR FATIGUE ** (CONT'D.)

Activity	Level of fatigue (1–10)
Reading	
Concentrating	
Housework	
Child care	
Making love	

Additional causes:

_____

_____

In addition to rating your fatigue triggers, it may be helpful to notice what time of day you have the most energy and what time you need to crash. When it comes to managing fatigue, you may have to budget your energy the way you budget your money.

Although resting doesn't work for everyone, I strongly suggest that you experiment and make time during the day for a nap. Napping is scientifically proven to enhance learning skills and cognitive abilities. Though still not widely practiced in this country, sleep researchers estimate that 40 to 60 percent of the world's adult population naps. These nappers can't all be wrong. Entire books have been written on the benefits of napping, even for those who don't suffer from illness. *Power Sleep*, by Dr. James B. Maas, and *Sleep to Save Your Life*, by Dr. Gerald Lombardo, both sing the praises of napping and are great resources if you are a novice napper.

How you approach your nap can be as important as the nap itself. Try to create a restful environment by lowering the lights, using earplugs, and finding a quiet spot. Make sure that you won't be interrupted by phone calls or visitors. It helps to set an alarm clock so that you're not worried about over-sleeping. You may not fall asleep, but you'll probably find that just resting in a quiet setting with your eyes closed can be restorative. Most of my clients report that if they rest during the day and heed the early warning signs of fatigue, they can avoid the self-defeating pattern of overdoing and recovering. Generally, a nap of thirty minutes to an hour seems to be enough rest to rejuvenate patients, although this will vary from person to person. Research shows that the minimum length of time needed to achieve a sleep that is actually restorative is about 20 minutes.

Making time for napping takes some creativity. One woman with small children says that she naps on the couch while the kids watch a video in the afternoon. Another mom arrives 30 minutes early to pick up her kids from school and closes her eyes until her children come pouring into the car. Some people bring a blanket and pillow to work and sleep in their cars during lunch. Others have made arrangements at work to have a cot or couch in a private room where they can retreat for a while.

Believe me, I understand how difficult it is to discipline oneself to rest. If taking a nap feels impossible, then take small breaks during the day. This may mean doing one thing at a time and then taking a short break before starting the next task. Often, you will be able to go on to the next activity within minutes and feel refreshed. One young MS patient says, "I've changed the way I manage my time. I've changed my priorities. I think twice before I commit to an activity, and I decide if it's something I really want or need to do." Getting proper rest often requires asking the question, "Is this something I need to do or something that would be nice to do?" Your answer may help you determine whether you should delegate errands to friends or family or make a social commitment.

Fatigue can often cause one's chronic symptoms to get worse. When wiped out, you may experience a recurrence of numbness, clumsiness, vertigo, blurry vision, or difficulty concentrating. An increase in muscle spasms or pain may occur. When my eyes begin to twitch, I know it is a physical signal for me to slow down and take a break. Just as in the case of stress, you must listen to your body and respect fatigue.

There have been times during deep fatigue when I had to stay in bed for a few days before feeling refreshed. Although I've never read any scientific evidence to support the idea that resting can avert an attack, I do believe I've been able to rest my way out of potential exacerbations, and I've heard many other patients report this experience as well.

In addition to resting, here are some other tips for conserving energy:

❖ Accept help when it is offered.

❖ Prioritize your tasks and get the most important chores done first.

❖ Learn to say "No."

❖ Apply for a handicapped parking permit and use it.

❖ Use a scooter at the mall or grocery store.

❖ Reduce stimulation by turning the TV or radio down or off.

❖ Shift expectations of yourself.

❖ Make time for what you like to do.

❖ Use lists and stay organized.

❖ Use delivery services for groceries or dry cleaning.

❖ Delegate.

❖ Don't wear high heels.

❖ Sit when you don't have to be standing.

❖ Use a wheelchair at the airport when you have to move from gate to gate.

❖ Take responsibility for the less physically demanding chores at home and assign the more difficult ones to other family members.

❖ Use adaptive devices.

❖ Take up less demanding hobbies like computer work, knitting, reading, puzzle solving, writing, and chatting on the phone.

❖ Only do things with small groups of people for short periods of time.

Let me address a couple of items on the above list that patients often seem resistant to.

In my experience, the suggestion to use adaptive devices can pose an extreme psychological barrier. Accepting that it is time to use a cane, leg braces, a scooter, or a wheelchair can represent a significant loss for patients. But the payoff can bring big gains. Countless times I've been told how the use of these tools has expanded and enriched the lives of patients. Gary, a man in his twenties with progressive MS, explains:

> It was painful to admit I needed to use a scooter. To me, it meant that my disease was really serious and could no longer be ignored. But using it got me out and into the world again. I was able to take my daughter down to the river and use the path to go for "walks." She and I would have some of our best talks when we got outside like that together. I'm sorry it took me so long to realize what I was giving up by resisting the help.

Patients are also often resistant to using handicapped parking permits. Some may feel embarrassed or ashamed about using these permits if they don't actually have to use an adaptive device. To make things worse, people are prone to making nasty comments when they see someone using a handicapped space who seems perfectly capable of walking. However, this is an energy-saving tool. If fatigue is one of your primary symptoms, it is completely acceptable for you to use the space. For those of you who experience symptoms after just a few moments in the sun, these spaces can also be a lifesaver when the weather is hot.

Nutrition

If we're going to talk about energy-sappers, we must not ignore the dreaded four-letter word—diet. When I was first diagnosed, the disease-modifying drugs that we have today were not yet available, so I looked for every possible alternative treatment I could find.

Initially, I tried a no-wheat, no-meat, no-sugar, no-dairy diet in order to rule out any allergies that might drain my immune system. I lost weight, but my MS didn't improve. I also went on the highly touted "low-fat Swank diet," a diet that was designed by Dr. Swank to reduce MS symptoms that was popular at the time. I lost weight, but my MS didn't improve.

Over the years, what I've learned is what science seems to bear out as true: Refined sugar is an energy drain on the system. When I cut down on sugar, my energy level went up. It even felt as if my sugar cravings went away and I was less likely to crash in the afternoons. I also started to add lean protein to every meal. This seemed to give me an energy boost as well. Eating four or five small meals a day also seems to increase stamina and regulate energy better than eating two or three larger meals.

Regardless of your health status, eating a balanced, healthy diet will surely make you feel better and improve your chances of fighting disease. The less weight you have to carry around, the less tired you will be. Try picking up a 10 or 20 pound weight and walking around with it. Imagine if you lost that amount? Experiment with what works best for you. Notice which foods drain you and which ones give you sustained energy (rather than candy-bar-type products that provide a quick pick-me-up that's sure to make you crash). Because diet is one of the few things we can control, it can give us a sense of mastery and confidence to eat well and feed our body fuel that helps us run at maximum efficiency. Ivy Larson, who has MS, and her husband, Dr. Andrew Larson, wrote a diet book, *The Gold Coast Cure*, which promotes a well-balanced healthy diet that is also intended to support the health of those with chronic illnesses. Talking to a nutritionist can help you get going on a healthy eating plan.

Exercise

At the risk of sounding repetitive, I must emphasize the importance of exercise one more time. Not only does regular exercise help reduce stress, it also increases energy, when performed with awareness and pacing. Traditionally, exercise has received little attention or emphasis in treating MS fatigue because physical activity was thought to exacerbate the condition.

However, recent research by Dr. Nadine Fisher at the State University of New York in Buffalo has shown that resistance exercise performed three times a week for one hour actually reduced fatigue—and increased endurance, speed, strength, and functional performance in MS patients. Those who maintain muscle tone exert less energy during the day when they do simple tasks such as lifting groceries or bathing a child.

Your exercise routine needs to be customized to meet your needs and abilities. You should consult a physical therapist to design the right program for you. A routine that helps you to maintain mobility (stretches) and increase endurance (weight lifting or swimming) is optimal. By interspersing periods of rest and recuperation, you should be able to find a fitness program that rejuvenates rather than exhausts you.

Your new exercise routine may be a very different type of workout than what you're used to. The goal is not necessarily to create a perfectly sculpted body, but to maintain good health and increase your energy throughout the day. This can be a difficult adjustment if you're used to a more rigorous workout program. Samantha, a 33-year-old MS patient, recalls:

> I used to train for triathlons. After my first serious attack, I had to completely change my mentality about working out. The running and swimming I had been doing were no longer an option. In the past, I worked out to stay competitive and that was my motivation. After MS, I had to learn to live with my limitations but still stay active. I overdid it many times and ended up exhausted for days at a time—eventually, I adjusted my expectations of what I could do and why I was doing it. Working with a knowledgeable trainer at my health club helped me design a new program that I was able to succeed at without wearing myself out.

Family Support

Family members can also be an integral part of your plan to help you manage fatigue. They may serve as a critical buffer, protecting you against exhaustion. With your input, loved ones can learn to be sensitive to important signals that indicate you've reached your fatigue saturation point. My husband says I become white as a sheet and expressionless when I've pushed myself too far.

You may want to develop a rating scale, such as the type you might use to describe pain, to let others know you're tired. On the scale, 1 would indicate feeling peppy and 10 would mean you're dog-tired and unable to go on.

In social situations I hate to always be the party pooper by saying we have to leave, so my husband and I have a signal that I give when it's time to go. I simply crook my index finger and he understands we need to take off pronto.

It's often necessary for family members and friends to help out and do extra work around the house. Delegating the more taxing chores can be imperative in managing fatigue. This can take skillful negotiation and a great deal of understanding from others. You may want to point out to those closest to you that they will directly benefit by helping you limit your fatigue. When we monitor and minimize our exhaustion, we can be more like our old selves: fun, silly, vibrant. When rested, we may once again feel like we have something left to give. We might even feel like making love! This is often a real incentive to get spouses to help out. If we avoid overdoing it, we can also reduce the likelihood of experiencing many of the chronic problems caused by MS that aren't only difficult for you, but no picnic for loved ones either.

Of course, no matter how sensitive our loved ones are to our needs, it's ultimately up to us to know when too much is too much. Since this can vary from day to day, it can be extremely hard for family members to monitor our energy level as well as we can.

Knowing that fatigue can make all other symptoms more intense is a great motivator to keep our commitments at a reasonable level and to allow ourselves time to recuperate.

Physical and Occupational Therapy

Your doctor may feel that physical or occupational therapies are warranted to help you manage your fatigue. Occupational therapy is particularly beneficial because these professionals are specifically trained to help you maintain your highest level of functioning. A good OT will find creative ways for you to still be productive and reach your optimal level of functioning within your limitations. Physical therapy can help you to learn new ways to improve your ability to move while using less effort, which in turn will save you energy. You may also learn of other ways to use adaptive devices to decrease physical exertion.

One patient with MS gives a great example of how she learned to minimize exhaustion:

> I still drive, although I don't do much more than go to the grocery store or doctor's office. I'd been driving to work, though, where I had to walk from the parking lot to my office. Since I live in Chicago, I would often have to scrape the ice off my windshield and I would freeze while waiting for the car to warm up. Plus, I had to make sure the driveway was plowed. I would be exhausted before I even got to my office. I started having the handicap van pick me up in the morning and return me home at night. It saved me the walk to and from the parking lot. Anything that helps me minimize the exhaustion is the way to go!

Anything that will minimize your exhaustion *is* the way to go. In your home, you might sit at a table while you chop veggies for dinner or set up a stool by the stove while you cook or always sit down when you talk on the phone. An occupational therapist can help you come up with many clever ideas that will fit your specific needs and situation in order to conserve energy.

Deep Breathing

Previously, I mentioned how deep breathing can help reduce stress and put you in a relaxed state; however, it can also give you energy. When we increase our oxygen intake, it can charge us up. Deep breathing is your internal organs' way of stretching. As your respiration becomes more active, your energy level rises. Deeper and fuller breathing gets oxygen to the brain and helps you feel more alert. When you're feeling sluggish, simply take four or five deep, full breaths and see if you notice a difference. You will have the best results if you can go outside to get fresh air. Follow this up by brushing your teeth and splashing water on your face. Most likely you will get a quick second wind. These steps are especially helpful following a nap, when you still feel a bit groggy.

Self-Honesty

One final thought about managing fatigue. Self-honesty may be one of the most effective ways to conserve energy. This life skill is the key to living with integrity. When you're true to yourself, you live without conflict. Tell the truth, and you live without guilt or fear. When your energy is not being used or depleted by living at cross-purposes, you're not draining yourself. If you're doing what you say you're going to do and you tell others what's in your heart, even if it's uncomfortable, a loosening will occur within your spirit. You will be free from second guessing yourself. By practicing self-honesty, you're liberated from the many unnecessary stresses that occur when we're less than straight forward about our intentions.

Self-honesty also means that you acknowledge your limits and honor your body when it needs rest.

Avoid the Mind-Reading Trap:

Sharpening Your
Communication Skills

I want my husband to know what I'm feeling. I want him
to be able to look at me, see how exhausted I am, and
know that I need him to fix dinner when he walks in
the door.

— Debbie; age 33, banker and wife, MS patient for 5 years

Any family therapist will tell you that lack of communication is
one of the most pressing problems in relationships. Unfortunately,
when chronic illness enters the picture, good communication becomes an even greater challenge. If families struggled to communicate prior to MS, patterns of nonproductive communication can
become intensified when the disease strikes. Lance Christensen is
former program manager for the Oregon chapter of the National
Multiple Sclerosis Society. He insightfully points out, "The greatest need of MS patients and their families is better communication. The root of many emotional problems is a lack of talking
openly with one another."

Since experts agree that keeping the lines of communication open may be the single most important factor in maintaining a healthy partnership, it's critical to learn the skills needed to effectively listen and be heard. Furthermore, by increasing your awareness of communication barriers, you may be able to minimize future conflicts.

The Mind-Reading Trap

The most frequent cause of misunderstanding among the clients I treat stems from the unrealistic expectation that a partner should automatically know what the patient wants, needs, or feels. This is an unfair demand that often leaves both parties disappointed and hurt. However, it's easy to understand how this desire arises. Living with our illness day-in and day-out, we become intimately aware of how we're feeling moment-to-moment, so shouldn't our loved one be aware as well? We desperately want them to be able to read our moods and physical abilities because so often we feel alone in our struggle.

Although we may cling to our wistful fantasy, the ability to mind read is an expectation that even the most devoted and loving partner will fail to meet. As you know, your disposition and physical abilities can vary throughout the day. Since many symptoms may be invisible, it's difficult for others to interpret what you may be going through. Unless you specifically express what you need or feel, more than likely, you will continue to be disappointed by those you love. Of course, expressing oneself isn't always an easy task. If it's your nature to hold things in or you're more of a giver than a taker, then asking for what you need may feel very uncomfortable. However, if you're to going to stay connected for the long haul, you must develop this ability.

By and large, the relationships that stand the test of time and endure crises are based on direct communication and trust. The next time you find yourself resenting your spouse or other family member for not understanding how you feel, describe for them what's going on. For example, if you have plans one night and don't feel up to going out, you might say, "I want to go out with our friends tonight, but this is one of my bad days and I know if I go I'll just feel pressure to be entertaining and I'll be lousy company. When we get home, I'll not only be more exhausted, but I'll feel badly about myself for seeming like a bore." The important thing is that you express what *you're* feeling. If you think your partner wants to get out, suggest that they go alone and catch you up on things when they come back. This may help you to feel less guilt or pressure to go to a party you would rather skip.

Hoping that your partner will "see" that you don't want to go out will rarely ever be effective. They won't necessarily "see" when you're too tired to make dinner or need help carrying things in from the car, either. The truth is, whether you have an illness or not, most people don't see what they don't want to. Others will assume that everything is normal and fine unless you tell them differently.

For years, I would get furious with my husband for keeping us out late at social gatherings. He loves to be the first to arrive and the last to leave. After MS fatigue took hold of me, his *joie de vivre* went from being one of the things I enjoyed most about him to one of the things I liked the least. I couldn't believe that he missed the yawns and evil glares I sent his way when I was tired. If he were looking for an excuse to go, he might have noticed my weariness, but he wanted to stay, so he ignored me. It wasn't until we started the signal of crooking my finger when it was time to go that this tension between us was resolved. Occasionally, we would take separate cars if I knew ahead of time that I was likely to want to leave a gathering before he would. This plan eased my guilt for escaping early. These were a few of the strategies we used to deal honestly and openly with my fatigue.

One MS patient would leave a sticky-note on the refrigerator for her husband to check when he got home. It would rate her feelings; good, bad, or terrible. These messages let her husband know what kind of day she was having and what she was up for that night. She liked this method because it helped her communicate without feeling as if she were complaining.

Family members often say that the greatest frustration of living with someone with MS is not knowing what to expect from
day-to-day. They want to know how their loved one is feeling and
they're usually willing to give them what they need, but often
they're left in the dark, trying to guess. Fred, the husband of one
MS patient says, "There are times when I can tell Beth is angry
with me, but she just goes on cooking or washing the dishes, bang-
ing things around. If I ask her what's wrong, she yells at me and
says, 'What do you think?' I honestly don't know. It just makes me
want to go into the other room and turn on the TV." After asking
Beth what was wrong, she typically exploded, "I needed your help.
I was exhausted. Couldn't you see that?" No. Fred couldn't see.
Beth had always been the one to handle the domestic chores in
their relationship. It never occurred to him to offer to wash the
dishes. He was willing to help, but he needed to know specifically
what Beth wanted and needed. Until they talked it through, Fred
just thought he had done something wrong and that Beth was angry with him.

The fluid nature of MS makes it even more difficult for family
members to know what is going on with the MS patient. On good
days, Beth was perfectly able to do the dishes and keep up with
housework. Fred had no way of knowing which days were good and
which were bad.

The next time you find yourself wishing that your loved ones
would just read your mind and know how you're feeling, take a moment to speak your feelings out loud and then ask for what you
need. It's always best to speak up before you reach your breaking
point. This could be the single most important thing you do to
improve your communication skills.

Accepting Help Can Be a Gift to Others

Another common obstacle to open communication is the fear of
becoming a burden. Once people become ill or fragile, they often
believe that others will quickly tire of hearing about how they feel
or assisting them with chores. While working as a home health so-

cial worker, I once made an early morning visit and found my client lying on the floor, writhing in pain. Through her tears she explained, "I could've reached the phone, but I didn't want to wake anybody at that hour. I knew one of you girls from the visiting nurses would be along eventually." It broke my heart to think that, rather than be an inconvenience, this elderly woman suffered needlessly for hours. Granted, this is an extreme example, but it illustrates the point that people will go to great lengths to avoid being considered a burden. This fear often shuts down communication.

"She never complained," people may wistfully recall when talking about their dearly departed grandmother. However, who knows how miserable Grandma might have felt inside as she endured her pain or disability under a cloak of lonely despair. What opportunities did her family miss to express their love and care for her while she bit her tongue and held in her needs? Could her life have been made richer and fuller had she let others come to her aid?

Accepting help from others is often a gift to them. It allows loved ones to feel needed and appreciated. To care for the needs of another affirms one's own value and purpose for living. Your vulnerabilities may teach a child empathy or help build a friend's self-esteem. When you allow another to run an errand or cook you a meal, you allow the best of the giver to shine. Recently, a patient told me the following story:

> For several years now, I've given myself a weekly injection of Avonex. Well, it had gotten to the point that my thighs needed a break so I asked my husband if he would give me a shot in the arm. (No pun intended.) I was worried about asking him because truthfully, he had fainted before at the doctor's office while giving blood and I just wasn't sure he could handle it. I didn't want him passing out while sticking me with a large needle. I also felt like I was giving up some control. I feel a great sense of independence by giving myself the shots. But the time had come. We both were nervous, and I almost changed my mind, but we did some mock trial runs, and then we just said the hell with it and went for it. To my surprise, I barely felt the needle go in. It was so much less painful than when I gave the

injection to myself. After it was over, he became very emotional and I asked him if it had freaked him out. He said, "No, it's just that this was the first time in the eight years since you've had MS that I could really do something to help you." It was really sweet. It made me realize how helpless *he* had been feeling.

This story illustrates that when we show our vulnerabilities, we're more likely to connect with each other. Letting others in to witness our pain or understand our needs makes us seem more approachable and human and, in short, more loveable.

Where Are We Coming From?

Women and men often see things from different perspectives and this disparity can cause a great deal of misunderstanding in relationships. John Gray, author of *Men Are from Mars, Women Are from Venus*, hit that nerve when he wrote a national bestseller concerning the differences in communication styles between men and woman. Clearly, there are variations in how men and woman convey their thoughts, feelings, and intentions. When we understand these gender differences, many misunderstandings can be avoided.

Women and men have different needs. A woman with a problem longs to be heard. We feel a great sense of relief as the words fall from our lips uninterrupted. We take comfort in simply getting our feelings out on the table, with a few nods of encouragement or consolation as a response. We want to feel a connection and be understood. In our eyes, a good listener is the sexiest companion imaginable.

Unfortunately, as Dr. Deborah Tannen points out in the book *You Just Don't Understand*, men are "fixers and protectors." Therefore, while a woman simply wants to hear, "I understand; you're not alone," what she may get instead is advice from her husband on how to solve her problem. Dr. Tannen gives the following example: "Eve had a lump removed from her breast. Shortly after the operation, talking to her sister, she said that she found it upsetting to have been cut into, and that looking at the stitches was distressing because they left a seam that had changed the contour of her breast. Her sister said, 'I know. When I had my operation, I felt the same way.' " Eve felt understood by her sister. But when she told her husband Mark the same thing, he said, "You can have plastic surgery to cover up the scar and restore the shape of your breast."

Mark's comment hurt her. Not only did she sense that her feelings were being discounted, she felt that he was asking her to go back under the knife at the very time she was explaining to him how much this surgery had upset her. Eve was comforted by her sister's validating response and injured by her husband's solution-focused comment.

On the other hand, men are sincerely baffled and frustrated by women's refusal to accept their help and advice. Dr. Tannen states that men perceive woman as wanting to wallow in their problems and talk about them forever, whereas men want to get their feelings out and either find a solution or laugh them off, so they can be done with them.

It's easy to see how this can cause many conflicts and misgivings—particularly when it comes to dealing with an incurable disease like MS. Many of the men I've talked with feel helpless and impotent when dealing with this disease. MS is not a broken pipe that can be repaired. When faced with the inability to protect their loved one or themselves from pain and disability, men feel like failures. Some women feel this way, as well.

The good news is that both husbands and wives can do something to comfort each other. They can learn to listen and be supportive. They can ask, "How can I help?" and they can try to be sensitive to their partner's moods.

Good communication is something that can be learned with practice, as long as there is a willingness to try.

Improving Communication: It's a Two-Way Street

Few of us are born gifted communicators. It's a skill that must be developed, just like competent writing or gourmet cooking. During my social work graduate program, we were taught a great deal about the nuances of effective communication; however, when you get down to it, there are two simple elements to good communication: listening and speaking. By gaining skills in both these areas, you will become a competent communicator.

Before learning more about how to improve your communication skills, take a moment to evaluate your current communication style. The exercise below will allow you to identify your speaking and listening strengths and weaknesses:

YOUR COMMUNICATION STYLE **

1. I often feel misunderstood.	True	False
2. People frequently interrupt me.	True	False
3. I feel anxious when speaking up for myself.	True	False
4. I let my partner do most of the talking for me.	True	False
5. I feel shy about asking for clarification when I don't understand what has just been said to me.	True	False
6. I find it easier to communicate through the written word.	True	False
7. It's hard for me to look people in the eye when I'm speaking.	True	False
8. I'm often told I don't listen well.	True	False
9. I get inpatient when others are talking.	True	False
10. When others are speaking, I'm often thinking more about how to respond to them than about what is being said.	True	False
11. I think talking is a waste of time.	True	False
12. I would rather do something about a problem than talk about it.	True	False

If most of your answers to questions 1–7 were true, there is a good chance that you need to increase your *speaking skills* and develop greater comfort in expressing yourself.

If most of your answers to questions 8–12 were true, learning to become a better *listener* will enhance your communication. Since communication is so important to our relationships and there are often many opportunities for misunderstandings when we have MS, it's worth investing some time to strengthen our communication skills. The fewer problems we have with communication, the less likely we are to feel frustrated or stressed and the less our body and energy are taxed. Here are a few suggestions on how you can improve your ability to communicate effectively:

IMPROVING YOUR SPEAKING SKILLS

Time your conversations. Choose to bring up an issue when you feel good and have the energy to handle it.

Try not to have conversations when your emotions are out of your control. That is not to say that you can't be angry, frustrated, or hurt—you just don't want to be so irrational and upset that you stop making sense.

Write out the major points you want to make before speaking.

Try not to use all-or-nothing statements such as "You never. . . " or "You always . . . . "

Take responsibility for expressing how *you* feel. Remember: Don't depend on "mind reading."

Maintain eye contact for at least 15 seconds at a time.

Ensure that no other distractions, such as the radio or television, are competing with your message.

Choose the right setting. You may find that talking while you're going for a walk or sitting outdoors relaxes you and makes conversation easier.

Avoid making personal attacks or using insults.

Be as direct and courteous as you can.

Avoid statements like, "You know what I'm saying." Be specific and say exactly what you mean.

Use feeling statements such as, "I feel that you get angry when I ask you to help around the house." Starting the conversation with "I feel" helps people respond less defensively, and it's a type of statement that can't be rationally refuted. You have a right to your feelings.

Realize that others may not always agree with you, but there is satisfaction in getting your message or feelings across. Yours may not be *the truth*, but it's your truth, and it's valid from your perspective.

Work on improving your confidence. Don't assume that what you have to say isn't worthwhile.

Keep in mind that the listener's silence doesn't imply consent or disagreement; they may just need time to process what they've heard.

Maintain an open mind. Be flexible about compromises or alternative solutions if you're discussing a problem.

Ask your listener to please reserve their comments until you get your point across, and then give them the same courtesy.

If you're discussing a touchy subject, you may want to start by saying that it's hard for you to have this conversation.

Check in with the person you're speaking to and ask if they've understood what you said.

As you begin to incorporate some of these suggestions into your conversations, you will begin to develop more confidence and feel misunderstood less often.

BECOMING A BETTER LISTENER

With so many competing demands needing our attention, it can be difficult to slow down and listen to our loved ones. To become a good listener, however, your focus needs to be entirely directed toward the speaker. Listening is not the same as hearing. You hear background noise. You listen to a friend. Listening is active. It means that you're making an effort to understand the perspective of the speaker.

In *On Becoming a Person*, psychotherapist Carl Rogers discusses the subtleties of listening:

> The whole task of psychotherapy is the task of dealing with a failure in communication. . . . The major barrier to mutual interpersonal communication is our very tendency to judge, to evaluate, to approve or disapprove the statement of the other person, or the other group. . . . Real communication occurs when we listen with understanding—to see the idea and attitude from the other person's point of view, to sense how it feels to them, to achieve their frame of reference in regard to the thing they are talking about.

Listening is becoming a lost art. It may be especially difficult to know how to listen if we weren't heard or acknowledged while growing up. Without role models to show us the best way to hear another person, we may feel at a loss to know how to respond when a loved one is trying to talk to us. However, everyone can elevate their listening skills. Below are a few suggestions for you to try out the next time someone you love is attempting to connect with you:

> Avoid interrupting. Let the other person finish their thought or make their point.

> Ask questions for further clarification: "So what you're saying is. . . ."

> Don't feel as if you have to respond right at that moment. If you need time to take in what you've heard, say, "Let me think about that."

Give the person your full attention. Turn your body toward the speaker, keep your arms uncrossed, and look them in the eye.

Resist the temptation to be distracted by other things, like paying bills or cooking.

Avoid framing a response while you're listening; instead, focus on listening.

Avoid giving suggestions and advice or trying to fix the problem.

Practice reading body language so that you can better understand the emotion behind the words that are being spoken.

Don't try to talk someone out of their feelings or discount their experience, no matter how painful it is to hear what they're saying.

Ask for clarification on the meaning of vague or unfamiliar terms.

Avoid making assumptions.

Ask open-ended questions to encourage further discussion.

Avoid expressing criticism or sarcasm.

Using these suggestions should instantly improve your listening skills. Recently, I came across a poem on the Internet written by an unknown author. It's a poignant reminder of how important it is to be a good listener:

When I ask you to listen to me, and you start giving me advice,
you have not done what I asked.

When I ask you to listen to me, and you begin to tell me why I
shouldn't feel that way, you are trampling on my feelings.

When I ask you to listen to me, and you feel you have to do
something to solve my problem, you have failed me, strange as
that may seem.

Listen! All I asked was that you listen, not talk or do—just
hear me.

*Advice is cheap; 20 cents will get you both Dear Abby and
Billy Graham in the same paper.*

*I can do for myself; I'm not helpless—maybe discouraged and
faltering, but not helpless.*

*When you do something for me that I can and need to do for
myself, you contribute to my fear and inadequacy.*

*But when you accept as a simple fact that I do feel what I feel,
no matter how irrational, then I can quit trying to convince
you and you can get about the business of understanding
what's behind this irrational feeling.*

*When that's clear, the answers are obvious and I don't need
advice.*

*Irrational feelings make more sense when we understand
what's behind them.*

*Perhaps that's why prayer works, sometimes, for some people—
because God is mute, and He/She doesn't give advice or try to
fix things. "They" just listen and let you work it out for
yourself.*

So, please listen and just hear me.

*And if you want to talk, wait a minute for your turn—and I'll
listen to you.*

If you love someone who has MS and you feel frustrated that you
can't do more for them, think of this poem and know that you can
always just listen. If you have MS and feel that you're no longer
able to give to others the way you have in the past, remember you
can always just listen. This may be the greatest gift anyone can
ever give.

Barriers to Communication

There are some common mistakes that can lead to communication breakdown. These behaviors are sure to have an immediate

and negative impact on a conversation and prevent others from
feeling safe when expressing their feelings. To improve communication you will want to avoid the following conversation stoppers:

* Moralizing

* Persuading, lecturing, instructing, and arguing

* Placing blame or judgment

* Using humor to make light of another's feelings

* Threatening or warning

* Changing the subject or going off on a tangent

* Telling someone you don't understand why they feel the
  way they do

* Telling someone that they're stupid or ridiculous to feel
  the way they do

* Placating or talking down to someone

* Drinking or using drugs before having a talk

These may seem like obvious obstacles to communication;
however, many people—especially couples and families—develop
extremely destructive communication patterns over the years.
These patterns may become so habitual that people often don't realize they're sabotaging their conversations.

When you want to be heard, *what* you say isn't nearly as important as *how* you say it. Studies show that communication is con-
veyed on three levels: words, voice/tone, and nonverbal clues. You
may be surprised to learn that nonverbal clues are 55 percent effective, tone of voice is 38 percent effective, and words are 7 percent effective in delivering a message to others. Being aware of the
way we present ourselves and how we use our body language can
greatly enhance our communication skills. For instance, if you're
smiling while you're trying to convey a serious concern, you're
sending a mixed message to the other person. The person notices
your smile, which dilutes the importance of your concern. Since

tone of voice can be used to enhance your message, you may want to monitor your voice quality. Are you speaking softly or forcefully? Is your voice high or low? Generally, an even, audible, and calm tone of voice is the most powerful way to express yourself.

Talking with Your Kids about MS

Parents are often conflicted and confused over how to talk with their children about MS. What you reveal to your children about your disease is a very personal decision and is different for every family. Your relationship with your child and knowledge of your child's needs factor into what is appropriate to disclose and what is best left unsaid.

In general, kids pick up on the emotional tenor or mood of the household. They sense when something is wrong, and this creates anxiety. If nothing is said about the subject, MS becomes the proverbial pink elephant in the room that everyone tip toes around and pretends is not there. Kids who are not given the facts may imagine the worst—just like adults. When you give your kids information, you validate their experience and acknowledge that something has changed.

Talking about your disease opens the door for your children to ask questions that they might have and gives you the opportunity to reassure them. By talking freely about your disease, you may help the child become more willing to talk about his or her own feelings. This isn't to suggest that you tell your children everything. You know your child and you are the best judge of how much he or she can understand and handle.

In her book *How to Help Children Through a Parents' Serious Illness*, Kathleen McCue suggests that you tell your children three things:

1. Tell them you are ill.

2. Tell them the name of your disease.

3. Tell them your best understanding of what may happen.

How much additional information you share is up to you; however, you may want to keep in mind a few further considerations when talking to your kids about MS:

❖ Keep your explanation as simple and age-appropriate as possible. For instance, "Mommy gets sick sometimes and needs to lie down and rest." Simplicity keeps misunderstandings and confusion to a minimum.

❖ Reassure your children that MS isn't contagious and they will not catch it.

❖ Let your kids know that they're not to blame for your disease.

❖ Explain that you will not die from this disease, but that on some days you will feel better than others.

❖ Encourage your children to ask questions. Let them know that MS is okay to discuss.

❖ When initially talking to your children about MS, try to remain as calm and confident as possible. Your attitude and delivery will greatly influence how your kids responds to the news. Be sure to let your children know that you're going to do everything you can to take care of yourself and of them.

Keeping your kids informed isn't the same as depending on them for emotional support. It can be tempting at times to use children as confidants, but this isn't advisable. It's unfair to ask a child to parent a parent. Instead, try to seek support from other adult family members, friends, or support groups rather than from your children. (More information on how to do this is presented in Chapter 11.)

Often, kids unconsciously feel responsible for making their parents feel sick. While she was learning to give herself an injection, a young mother told me this story: "I hate the thought of giving myself a shot, but I have to do this. The other day I overheard my kids praying to God to make them behave well so that they wouldn't make me sick. It tore me up." Be sensitive to this type of reaction, and reassure your child that they are not the cause of your symptoms.

So how much *do* you reveal to your child? If you're on a medication that requires injection, should you let your children see you giving yourself a shot? Again, this depends on the age of the children. Keep in mind that it can be frightening for a child to walk in on a parent sticking their body with a needle. Explaining why you give yourself the shot, and letting your children know that the medicine is supposed to help you feel better, can be a great comfort. Some families even have their older children administer the injection. The famous country singer Clay Walker recently appeared on the *Larry King* show, and he told the audience that his children routinely give him his shot.

Typically, children want to help out when a parent becomes ill. In fact, it may be necessary for children to take over some of the household chores. Try to be specific about how your children can help the family and let them know that they're appreciated.

The National MS society provides a couple of brochures geared toward helping young people understand MS. By using illustrations and straightforward language, these pamphlets can assist you in explaining the disease to your children. You will find these listed in the Resource section of this book.

⌘ ⌘ ⌘

With the new skills you've learned in this chapter, you will be better prepared to discuss issues that are important to you with those you love. It will take practice to incorporate these techniques into your communication style, so be patient and don't give up. If you continue to have difficulty getting your message across, consider going to family therapy. Family therapists are mediators who can help you identify barriers to your communication and make suggestions on how to change unproductive patterns.

Staying Connected:

Improving Support Networks and Enhancing Intimacy

*The only thing that's gotten me through the
unpredictability of this disease has been the
dependability of my friends.*

— Karen; age 27, bank teller, MS patient for 2 years

Trying to deal with MS in a vacuum is difficult. Developing and maintaining healthy relationships with friends and family members is important for everyone, but if you have MS, it's paramount to managing the disease. However, staying connected to your loved ones when you have a chronic illness isn't always easy.

Illness challenges us to strike a balance between solitude and connectedness, between independence and interdependency. It makes us realize on a very basic level that we need others, and yet it requires us to take care of ourselves as best we can. Disability forces us to recognize which bonds will withstand the demands of disease and which ones won't. Since having a chronic illness can strain relationships, we must work hard to hold on to those we love and those who love us. Hold on for dear life.

Avoiding Isolation

Initially, people may try to hide their diagnosis from others as they struggle to adjust and come to terms with their disease. Fear of being stigmatized or seen as disabled may force patients into secrecy. Others may not mention their disease for fear of worrying or upsetting friends and family. Often, people with MS keep quiet and don't reach out because they feel it's impossible for others to understand what they're going through, but hiding an MS diagnosis only makes us feel even more isolated and disconnected. Mandy, a 37-year-old mother, says, "When I needed my friends and family the most, I shut them out. I thought that I could protect my teenage son by keeping my disease to myself. I was afraid if I told anyone, it would get back to my son and he would fall apart. It wasn't until I started dropping things and walking strangely that I told him. It turned out he was relieved. He thought that I was hiding a drinking problem!" Mandy's story is not unusual. When we keep those we love in the dark about our disease, they often suspect the worst. We must be honest with our families about our illness before they can support us and begin to understand our challenges.

Frequently patients feel socially isolated when living with a chronic illness. Depending on your level of disability, the challenge of simply leaving the house may become a hindrance to connecting with others. Fatigue can rob us of the motivation to shower, dress, and prepare to venture outside. If we can no longer drive, transportation becomes a complication that we must contend with. Using a walker or wheelchair can make it seem just too difficult to get out the door. Eventually, we may become withdrawn. We can get to the point where it no longer feels like going out is worth the effort. But it is.

The support of family and friends often gets us through tough times. Studies now show that there is a powerful motivation for staying socially active. Maintaining social contact is necessary for both mental and physical health. According to the CDC (Centers for Disease Control and Prevention), there is a strong correlation between having loving and supportive relationships and the ability to cope with illness and poor health. Compared with single, divorced, or widowed people, married men and women, or those in committed relationships, have longer lives, more monitoring of health, more compliance with medical regimes, and less depression, less stress, and less loneliness. Furthermore, married people in positive relationships with their spouses also show better heart and blood pressure responses to stress, and improved immune function. Research is proving that healthy relationships appear to make for more healthy bodies.

Whether it be a marriage, a partnership, a friendship, or simply a social acquaintance, being around others is good for us. Matt, a 48-year-old lumber broker, found friendship to be his salvation:

> I'd been divorced for a good six years prior to my diagnoses. We didn't have kids and my wife was sort of in charge of our social life. When we parted ways, many of my friends left, too. Work became my life. Then when I got MS, I realized that I had no one to depend on. It was frightening to feel so alone. I decided to move to an adult community. We all have our own apartments, but there is also a common swimming pool and lodge. Several of us play cards once a week and I've gotten to know many of my neighbors. We have each other over for dinner and sometimes throw parties. These people aren't family, but I feel like I can count on them if I'm in a pinch. It's reassuring to have people close by.

Because MS can put such tremendous demands on family members and friends, particularly when the patient needs physical care, it's extremely beneficial to enlarge your support network. Caregivers can burnout, but when the care is shared among others, this can be prevented. Chronic illness specialist, Gary Gilles, LCPC, says, "As a general rule, the more people you have involved in your life, the more effective you will be in managing both the emotional and physical aspects of your chronic medical condition." Although it may seem easier to depend solely on your closest contacts, it's important to make the effort to develop your social network and meet new people. The more people you have in your life, the less dependent you will be on just one person to meet all your needs. The support of friendships and family can truly have a huge impact on your quality of life with MS.

Sometimes we're unaware of the friendship and support that is available to us until we begin to reach out. This next exercise will help you identify the people and community resources that you can currently draw upon for companionship.

The Wheel of Support

On an 8½" x 11" sheet of paper, draw a circle two inches in diameter. Then write the name of the person you feel closest to in the center of the circle. Then draw another circle about an inch apart around the first circle. Now write the names of the three people you feel next closest too within that circle. Then draw a third circle, about an inch apart, around the second circle. Write the names of five people you could call on to ask a favor from in that circle. Now draw a fourth circle, about an inch apart, around the third circle. Write the names of any groups or clubs you belong to within that circle.

Finally, draw a fifth circle around the fourth circle and write in any community organizations that you could potentially call upon for services or support. If you're unfamiliar with the community resources in your area, you can refer to the Resources section in the back of this book to learn more about services that might be available to you.

This exercise can help you clearly visualize how much support you have access to when you're willing to ask for it. If you had difficulty identifying social supports, this may be an indication that you need to make a conscious effort to expand your network of relationships. That's the topic of the next section.

Making Connections

Many of us feel daunted by the task of making new acquaintances or joining groups. We may feel that our illness limits our ability to make new connections. Perhaps you are limited, but if there is a will, there is a way. Kelly, a 63-year-old widow and MS patient who could no longer walk without assistance, found herself feeling very isolated and alone after her husband died. She depended on neighbors and cabs to get her to appointments and she used a grocery delivery service for supplies. With some encouragement, Kelly called her local MS society to find out what types of services were available in her area. Initially, she thought she might attend a support group; however, after learning about the telephone peer support group, she decided to become a volunteer: "I'd lived with the disease for so long, I thought I might be able to share my experiences and help out new folks. It turns out I have a lot to offer them and they have a thing or two to teach me. I get the contact I need without having to leave my apartment."

There are a variety of ways to meet others and get the social stimulation you need; a few suggestions are given below.

WAYS—AND PLACES—TO MEET OTHER PEOPLE

Ask your local library if they have a book club you can join, or start one yourself.

Join a health club and take classes. It's no coincidence that exercise is suggested as a remedy for depression, fatigue, and isolation. Exercising with others can meet many needs.

Take a class at your local community college.

Explore MS chat rooms online (see the Resources section) and e-mail friends.

Call your local MS society and ask about support groups.

Explore volunteer opportunities.

Set a regular phone date with a friend.

Offer to pet-sit for others.

Make the effort to invite friends out, or in, for dinner.

Become active in a church or other spiritual program.

Find a friend who loves movies and have a regular movie night date.

Visit a nursing home.

Take a part-time job.

Get two season tickets to the symphony or a ball game and invite a guest each time.

Remember birthdays and invite your friends to lunch on those days.

Participate in your local community theatre.

Baby-sit for friends or relatives.

Look up old acquaintances and re-kindle friendships.

Attend a lecture series.

Visit a museum. (Venues such as museums often have wheelchairs available on-site to minimize the fatigue of walking and standing.)

Of course this list isn't all-inclusive, but it gives you an idea of the wide array of opportunities for you to connect with others.

MS Support Groups: Give Them a Chance

Talking with someone else who has MS can feel like coming home on a cold winter day and being wrapped in a warm blanket. The validation that comes from hearing another MS patient say, "I know what you mean," helps us feel normal and completely understood. Although our symptoms may differ, we all know what it feels like to experience a relapse, deal with treatment decisions, and live day-to-day with a chronic illness.

On several occasions I've had the opportunity to speak to MS support groups. The camaraderie that develops between the participants can be a lifeline for those who are feeling lost, lonely, or misunderstood. I've witnessed many deep friendships develop that extend beyond the confines of the group. The sharing of information and experience is valuable, yet the opportunity for emotional connections is priceless.

Despite all the benefits, clients are often resistant when I suggest that they attend these groups. The fear of seeing other MS patients with more advanced symptoms scares some people away. However, usually if I can convince a client to attend one meeting, they return singing the praises of the group. Give yourself the same chance and go to at least one meeting. Your local MS Society can provide you with information about what types of groups are available in your area (see the Resources section). Some local chapters have started offering support groups for various levels of disability as well as for people who are newly diagnosed. Kit and Susan met at one of these groups several years ago. Susan says:

> I had MS for many years before I went to my first MS support group. I had gone to an MS conference and met a few other gals there who also had MS. After realizing how good it was to talk with them, I finally decided to give my local group a try. Not being a group person, I was nervous. During my first meeting, a friendly little redhead came up to me, stuck her hand out, and said, 'I'm Kit and I'm glad you're here.' That was 10 years ago. Since then we've been through divorces, deaths of loved ones, job changes, health problems, you name it. We're always there for each other through good and bad. When we are going to get together, if I need to cancel plans because I'm having a bad day or I forget something she's told me, she understands. I don't know what I'd do without her.

Because other MS patients really "get it," these types of friendships are special indeed.

In addition to providing companionship, research shows that support groups lower levels of anxiety, increase positive feelings about social supports, teach coping skills, give techniques to manage specific symptoms, and promote health. These positive benefits are hard to pass up.

However, if attending a support group is just not your cup of tea, or if you're unable to physically get to a group meeting, the Internet now offers a variety of online support options. Chatrooms, message boards, websites, and discussion groups can all give you access to information and support right at your fingertips. (See the Resources section for a listing of online sites that can get you connected to others who have MS.)

Judith Nichols, author and MS patient, wrote a wonderful book about Internet friendships entitled *Women Living with MS*, which is based on her experiences in creating a support group online. Through her story you may find the inspiration you need to access the incredible resources waiting for you in cyberspace. Additional online support can be found by going to Google.com and searching "Multiple Sclerosis Support Groups." With so many options out there, you're certain to find a supportive connection that's right for you.

Intimacy Issues

If you're in a long-term relationship, then you know that sexual passion can ebb and flow. Everyday stresses and demands often place physical intimacy on the back burner, where it can get cold. It's common for everyone, with or without MS, to occasionally experience sexual difficulties. However, for people with MS, many additional hurdles can get in the way of having a satisfying sex life. Up to 90 percent of men and 70 percent of women with MS report having some type of sexual dysfunction. This isn't to say that you should no longer expect to experience sexual pleasure just because you have MS; it just means that you may have to address your specific issues and discover new ways to enhance your sexual experience. This section aims to help you do that.

CAUSES OF SEXUAL DYSFUNCTION

There are several causes of sexual problems that are specific to people with MS. Both physical and psychological issues may create sexual dysfunction. Physically, MS can impair the central nervous system. This means that the nerves connecting to the reproductive organs can get interrupted, slowing arousal time, reducing sexual desire, causing impotence, and interfering with the ability to have an orgasm. Other physical causes of sexual problems can arise from pain or lack of sensation, medication side effects, bowel and bladder changes, spasticity, and cognitive impairments. Psychologically, feelings of fatigue, low self-esteem, and depression can also cause one's sex drive to diminish.

Although it can be awkward, couples should make every effort to discuss their sexual difficulties. If you simply shy away from physical intimacy or avoid sex, your partner may assume you're no longer interested in them and not realize that MS-related physical or emotional problems are to blame.

Physical distance often leads to emotional distance, which is hurtful to both parties. Clay, a 42-year-old MS patient, began to have difficulty getting an erection. After he had tried to make love to his wife Mary a few times and was unable to perform, he felt ashamed and embarrassed. Rather than addressing the issue, he simply stopped making advances toward her. Mary couldn't understand why her husband was rejecting her. She began to feel undesirable and wondered if Clay still loved her. Clay and Mary ended up coming to counseling because Mary was contemplating having an affair. This is not an uncommon response when sexual relations cease in a marriage. After a few sessions, Clay revealed the physical problems he was having and this allowed us to begin discussing possible solutions. With medical treatment, he was able to once again sustain an erection. The physical problem was relatively easy to take care of, but it took a great deal of work for the couple to overcome the emotional pain that was caused by feelings of rejection and sexual withdrawing.

SEX SOLUTIONS

MS is no reason to abandon your sex life. Once sexual issues are brought out into the open, couples can begin to work through them and enjoy intimacy again. As we've discussed, emotional issues such as depression can be treated with medication and/or counseling. Impotency can also be treated with medications such as Viagra or Levitra. If fatigue is an issue, changing the time of day that you have sex can help increase desire. The use of lubricants, such as Astroglide or K-Y Jelly, and vibrators can be helpful for women who have difficulty with vaginal dryness or achieving orgasm. Emptying your bladder before sex can help you relax and avoid discomfort.

Talk with your doctor about any sexual concerns you're having. Communicating with your health-care professional is especially important since some of your problems may be successfully treated with medication. If you're uncomfortable talking with your doctor about sexual issues, write down a list of your problems and give it to your health-care provider to review.

Creativity, a sense of humor, fantasy, and flexibility will carry you a long way as you explore new approaches to your sexuality.

I often advise couples to experiment with ways to express their sexual needs that aren't genital focused. You and your partner may want to agree that you won't even attempt reaching an orgasm or having intercourse for a few weeks. Sometimes, teasing and foreplay are a great way to rekindle the spark. Try just kissing and touching each other without removing any of your clothing. Remember how passionate you felt when you were first getting to know your partner, but hadn't actually had sex? Re-creating this experience can be a wonderful way to encourage intimacy and recharge your libido.

If you're a man and impotency is an issue, try oral stimulation or a use a vibrator to satisfy your partner. Take the focus off the erection and put it toward pleasing your lover in other ways. Keep in mind that pleasing each other may not necessarily mean achieving an orgasm. Hugging, cuddling, or giving each other a massage or foot rub can be satisfying and erotic. You and your partner are in control of how you want to connect and feel intimate. Simply looking into your beloved's eyes and reaching out to hold their hand can be all one needs to feel loved and desired.

It's also helpful to let your partner know how and where you like to be touched. Don't hesitate to say what feels good. MS symptoms can change the way your body responds to stimulation. Your physical desires and pleasures may be different now and you will need to let your lover know what he or she can do to please the new you.

Of course, first *you* must know how you want to be touched. In the brochure *MS and Intimacy*, published by the National Multiple Sclerosis Society, the following body mapping exercise is recommended to help you rediscover your own body. Initially you'll want to do this exercise by yourself. By learning how to make yourself feel good, you will then be able to tell your partner what you enjoy.

BODY MAPPING EXERCISE*

* Excerpted from MS and Intimacy *with permission from the National Multiple Sclerosis Society. For more information call 1-800 FIGHT MS (1-800-344-4867).*

Begin this exercise in self-exploration with curiosity and an open mind. Be sure that you're in a comfortable setting where you won't be interrupted and give yourself about 15 minutes. To map out your personal bodily sensations, begin by gently touching yourself from head to toe. Take your time and notice what makes you feel pleasure as well as discomfort. Experiment with what feels good. What feels different? Are you numb in any area? Just take a few minutes to get to know yourself and your body at this moment in time. Repeat this exercise a few times a week. Allow yourself to feel pleasure, but don't focus on achieving an orgasm, as this may interfere with fully exploring all of the areas you enjoy having touched.

As you become more comfortable, you can include your partner in this exercise. Talk to each other during this exercise and tell each other what feels good and what feels better. Again, avoid focusing on reaching an orgasm. This exercise can help you rediscover each other and take your feelings of intimacy to a deeper level. Shelly, an MS patient who has been married for 17 years, describes her experience with body mapping:

> At first I was uncomfortable with the whole idea of it. But for years my husband and I had had a wonderful sex life, and then after a while it became nonexistent. This worried me. I felt like we were drifting apart. We had to do something. The MS did

make my body respond differently to touch. Some parts of my legs were numb and when we made love, the numbness seemed to get worse. Also, I couldn't tolerate the same amount of stimulation that I used to enjoy during sex. Instead of saying anything, I just started to avoid sex altogether. The mapping exercise helped me describe what was going on with me physically and to talk to my husband about it. We were able to start making some adjustments and learn more about what we both enjoy. Sex is back in our lives now and I think in some ways it's better than before.

Having sex is an important way for us to show our love and affection for each other, and when we neglect our sex life, our relationships invariably suffer. Although many people may feel uncomfortable when they first begin the body mapping exercise, the reward of increased physical intimacy is usually well worth the effort.

MAKING ROOM FOR ROMANCE

We all need to make room for romance in our lives; everyone gets in a rut from time to time. When this happens, it's time to shake things up with some spontaneity. This can be fun. Setting one night aside as a date night is a good way to spice up your love life. Make the evening special and be sure that the focus is just on each other. No kids or friends can be included. Do something fun and out of the ordinary. Go for a picnic at a local lake or beach, get an ice-cream sundae, take a walk in the woods, or attend a concert in the park. If you want to stay at home, make a candle-lit dinner, play romantic music, and slow dance together. This would be a great time to practice your listening skills. Really take an interest in your partner. Ask questions about how they're doing and what they're feeling. Slow things down so that for a few hours the world is just about the two of you.

SEX IS ALL IN YOUR HEAD

It's often said that sex is more about what happens above the belt than below it. Our thoughts and feelings are what drive us sexually.

It's not unusual for someone with MS to lose touch with their sexuality as they battle physical challenges. If your self-image changes due to illness and your self-esteem suffers, you may no longer feel like a sexual being. When this happens, your sex drive can falter and you will need to take some extra steps to get yourself recharged. Talking with your partner about your insecurities and the changes that may be going on with you is a good first step toward jump-starting your love life. Give your partner the chance to reassure you and express how much he or she still desires you. Hearing that you are wanted is a potent aphrodisiac.

Since much of our sexual motivation originates in our mind, the use of fantasy can often help stimulate sexual desire. Reading romance novels or watching sexy movies may be just what you need to get aroused. If you want a little inspiration, check out the book *101 Nights of Grrreat Sex: Secret Sealed Seductions for Fun Loving Couples*, by Laura Corn. This book is full of creative ideas to get your imagination going.

When we become disconnected from our physical selves, our sex life shuts down. If you've ignored your appearance and let yourself go, you may want to work toward getting back into shape. Guys, take the time to shave; gals, put on some makeup and style your hair. Wear something that makes you feel attractive. When you feel better about your appearance, you feel sexier.

WHEN YOUR LOVER IS YOUR CAREGIVER

"My husband sees me as someone he needs to take care of. He has become more like a parent than a lover. I already have parents. I need to feel like a woman again," says Anne, a 53-year-old housewife who has lived with MS for 20 years.

A common dilemma for spouses who are also caregivers is how to transition from one role to the other. When you're helping a loved one with daily activities, such as bathing or dressing or walking, it can be difficult to then see them as a lover or sexual being as well. Frequently, the patient who requires a great deal of physical care falls into a dependent role and the caregiver does become more like a parent. This can cause both parties to experience sexual confusion. Caregivers, particularly men, may fear hurting their partner or making their symptoms worse during love-making, so they avoid making sexual overtures in an effort to "protect" their loved one. Again, these issues need to be discussed and worked through.

Couples who successfully maintain the roles of lover as well as caregiver tend to keep their lives balanced. For instance, they do activities together that have nothing to do with MS. This helps to remind couples that they're partners and that each has something of value to offer the relationship.

Hiring a home-health aide or asking a relative or friend to help with some of the more intimate caregiving responsibilities, such as bathing and dressing, can help both partners preserve separate identities, which can reduce stress, resentment, and burnout.

When couples recognize that MS is a medical issue that needs to be dealt with, not a problem that defines the relationship, they're more likely to relate to each other as equals and maintain a healthy sexual relationship.

How you interpret your sex life is up to you and your partner. You're free to reinvent your sexual relationship so that it feels right for you both. The important thing is that you maintain trust and physical intimacy on some level and continue to talk about sexual issues when they arise.

If you continue to struggle with intimacy issues, you might want to consider seeking couples counseling to address the problem. Family therapists are generally well trained and prepared to assist couples who are struggling with sexual problems.

chapter
twelve

Coping with Cognitive Challenges

I don't know if my family has any idea how difficult it is
for me to think clearly and remember things. I'm too
scared to tell anybody because they might not view me
as the same person I used to be.

— Connie; mother of two, MS patient for 11 years

In some instances, cognitive issues may be more difficult for people to discuss than sexual problems. To admit that you're having
trouble remembering, understanding, and processing information
can be very frightening. Suddenly, you become vulnerable to the
judgments and assumptions others may make about your competency. You may risk losing your job or your responsibilities at home
if you reveal how muddled your mind can get. What is worse, you
begin to doubt yourself. Living with the secret knowledge of cognitive challenges can be a heavy burden to lug around. Trying to
cover for mistakes, second-guessing your own decisions, or going
mute when asked a question you can't answer can be very stressful.
However, if you suffer from cognitive changes, you're not alone in
your struggle.

It's estimated that between 45 and 65 percent of all MS patients experience some type of cognitive impairment. These challenges include problems with memory, attention, word-finding, problem solving, or slowed processing. The severity of cognitive changes can vary from one person to the next, and this type of problem can come and go just like any other MS symptom. Cognitive deficits can worsen during exacerbations or at times of extreme fatigue but then improve during remission or with rest. The unpredictability of our mental capabilities can cause even more confusion and frustration for both patients and family members.

To make matters more perplexing, just like with fatigue, there is little relationship between the severity of other physical symptoms and cognitive functioning. One person may have extreme physical disability and be sharp as a tack, while another may seem fine physically, but be unable to follow directions or read a book because they forget the sentence they just read. Fortunately, the majority of us will only experience mild to moderate deficits that we can learn to manage through compensating techniques.

In order to learn how to manage cognitive issues, you will first need to identify what types of cognitive problems pertain to you.

Types of Cognitive Challenges

According to Dr. Darcy Cox, a neuropsychologist at the University of California-San Francisco Multiple Sclerosis Center, there are seven distinct categories of cognitive deficits that MS patients may face. After reading this section, try to determine if you've experienced trouble in any of these areas.

MEMORY

There are actually two kinds of memory functions. The first is *procedural memory*. Procedural memory helps you to remember how to do things. Typically, this ability remains unchanged in people with MS. For instance, you may forget where your keys are, but you won't forget what they are for or how to use them.

The second memory function is *semantic memory*. This part of our memory allows us to remember events, words, names, or objects. This is the area of memory that is most likely to be impacted by MS. There are actually three parts to *semantic memory*:

❖ First, you must be able to pay attention to information and take it in. If you're having trouble with concentration, you won't be able to attend to information. When this occurs, you're not able to encode or learn new information.

❖ Learning and encoding information is the second aspect of semantic memory. If you're unable to take this step, it makes it harder to remember new phone numbers, appointments, directions, names, and new skills; however, you may be able to remember obscure names from the past with no problem because you learned these names before your brain was affected by the disease.

❖ Finally, you must be able to retrieve or recall information when you need it. For instance, we recently moved and I've met many new people in the area, but when I run into them for the third or fourth time, and I really want to remember their names, I draw a blank. This is an embarrassing problem, as you can imagine. The ability to recall this type of information has just vanished.

You may have difficulties in all three of these memory categories, or only in one or two. Depending on what part of your brain is impacted, you may be able to remember what you see but have problems remembering what you hear. By paying attention to where your strengths and weakness are, you can compensate by making adjustments in your learning style. For instance, if you're better at taking in information verbally and you need to learn something new, it may be better to listen to the information on tape rather than trying to read it from a book.

PROCESSING SPEED

Often MS patients experience an overall slowing in their ability to process information. For example, if someone is trying to show you how to download music onto your computer for the first time, you may need to have them explain it to you several times because you're only able to absorb one instruction at a time. It may take you a while to let the concept sink in before you can move on to the next task.

If you have this experience, give yourself permission to ask questions and to slow down the learning process. Just because you process information slowly, doesn't mean that you can't learn new skills. Tell the person providing you with the information that you need to go gradually. It can be tempting to pretend that you understand rather than asking for what you need, but when you do this, you miss out on more than is necessary. Be patient with yourself and ask others to do the same.

ATTENTION AND CONCENTRATION

Generally, people with MS are able to maintain attention during simple tasks; however, as the difficulty of the task increases, problems with concentration and attention increase. You may find that when you need to multi-task in the office or at home with children running around, you get frustrated and need to break activities down into one task at a time. In my case, I find that having the radio playing in the background while I'm trying to talk on the phone can feel overwhelming. I get irritated and feel an urgent need to shut the music off.

When you understand your own cognitive limitations, you can take measures to create an optimal working environment that allows you to be productive and feel less stressed.

COGNITIVE FATIGUE

As I've mentioned before, people with MS can get fatigued from doing mentally challenging work, even if they're not exerting themselves physically. Once you become cognitively fatigued, you're more likely to work slowly and make mistakes. For instance, the other day I was having a busy morning and by 9:00 A.M. I was already feeling overwhelmed. The next thing I knew, instead of pouring milk over my cereal, I was pouring the hot water for my tea over it.

When you become either mentally or cognitively fatigued, your existing physical and cognitive issues can worsen. For example, you may find that after concentrating for a few hours and working at the computer, your eyes begin to blur and your attention span shortens. This is a warning sign to take a break.

LANGUAGE

The most common language problems for MS patients include having difficulty in finding words and in naming things or people. When you're in the right mood, these faux pas can sometimes be good for a laugh. The other day we were at the grocery store I asked my husband to bring me a "carriage." "Yes your highness," he replied. He knows me well enough to realize that I was asking for a shopping cart but couldn't find the name for it. We both burst out laughing.

If the name of an object just won't come to you, you may need to draw upon your descriptive skills to explain or describe the word or the thing that has "flown away" for the moment. For instance, you may call your refrigerator "the thing that keeps food cold," or you may call a pot "the cooking thing." Often, as soon as you stop trying to find the word, it suddenly appears.

PROBLEM SOLVING

Sometimes MS patients have difficulty solving problems in new situations. When presented with a problem, you may try the same solution over and over again, rather than looking outside the box for a different approach. Decision making may become difficult, as you try to decide what choice is best. When you're faced with this issue, try walking away from the problem for a while and taking some time to think it over. You may find that with a good night's rest, new answers will come to you.

VISUAL AND SPATIAL SKILLS

People with MS can find themselves getting lost more frequently, misplacing things more often, or having difficulty understanding visual information such as maps, diagrams, and charts. Once I left a friend's party and went for a walk, just to get away from the noise and chaos for a few moments. I'd intended to walk around the block and come right back. Somehow I became completely disoriented and got lost. I didn't know the address of the home and panicked. This only made me more confused. Almost an hour later, to my great relief, I miraculously came upon their house once again. That experience shocked me and rocked my self-confidence. If you've had these "lost in space" moments, you can compensate for visual and spatial deficits by writing directions down or taking them verbally, rather than relying on a map or visual memory. Always have the physical address and phone number of where you're going and, most importantly, don't panic.

The Benefits of a Cognitive Evaluation

After considering these descriptions, if you suspect that you might have cognitive problems, and you haven't already addressed the issue, call your neurologist and set up an appointment to discuss any changes you've noticed.

Perhaps you're still questioning whether or not you have a cognitive deficit. If you're in doubt, ask a family member or trusted friend if they've noticed any difference in your thinking skills. Getting a second opinion may give you a more objective perspective. My husband always seems more aware of my memory problems than I am. Could denial be playing a role in my lack of awareness? Sure. None of us really wants to admit that we're having these issues, but like all symptoms related to MS, the sooner you start to deal directly with your concerns, the sooner you can begin to do something positive to improve your situation.

When you go in to see your physician, the doctor may ask if your problems are interfering with your ability to work or perform normal daily activities. If the answer is yes, they may recommend a neuropsychological evaluation. This is a fancy name for a series of tests that help determine the extent of your problem and identify the specific areas where you're having trouble. The tests also show where you continue to have strengths. In some instances, an evaluation may be used to determine if you're able to continue working. This type of evaluation may be required if you're applying for disability benefits. Although not widely recognized, cognitive difficulties can often interfere with one's ability to work even more than physical problems.

One word of caution: Your insurance may not necessarily pay for this test, and it can be expensive. Check with your insurance company ahead of time to determine what part of the cost it will cover, so that you know how much you'll have to pay out-of-pocket.

If you're about to start one of the disease-modifying drugs, this can also be a good time to consider getting an evaluation so that you can obtain a baseline of your cognitive functioning. The baseline will allow you to track changes that occur over time and to determine whether or not the drug is effective in treating your cognitive problems.

Knowing what your cognitive strengths and weaknesses are will enable the doctor to develop a concrete plan of action to help you compensate for your deficits. For instance, if memory problems are caused by difficulty concentrating, strategies may be recommended to reduce distractions so that it becomes easier for you to concentrate. If, on the other hand, your memory problems are caused by difficulty retrieving information, you may be encouraged to develop a system to increase your use of reminders.

When you don't realize the cause of your cognitive changes, you can literally feel like you're losing your mind. Family members may become irritated with your memory lapses, employers may question your competency, and friends may feel that you just don't care enough to remember the details of their lives. These misunderstandings can be extremely painful and stressful. A neuropsychological evaluation may explain why you have these cognitive problems, and it can validate your experiences. The results you receive from an evaluation can go a long way toward improving your self-esteem and repairing relations with others.

Cognitive Therapy

Once an evaluation has been completed, your doctor may recommend cognitive rehabilitation therapy. Generally, a neuropsychologist or occupational therapist can perform cognitive rehabilitation as long as you have a doctor's referral.

Similar to physical therapy, cognitive therapy normally requires an hourly session once a week for several weeks depending on your individual needs. In these sessions you will be taught "compensatory strategies" to combat cognitive issues. These might include organizational skills, computer skills, and time-management techniques. You may also have to do exercises to improve memory, concentration, or spatial skills. Although cognitive rehabilitation doesn't treat the underlying impairment, it can improve your functioning and quality of life. In addition, cognitive therapy can help family members to better understand the cause of specific problems, and it often encourages them to learn more about how they can assist you.

Medication for Memory

Unfortunately at this date, few medications have been found to help treat memory problems. However, Avonex, one of the MS disease-modifying drugs mentioned earlier, did show modest benefits for a variety of cognitive functions in one large clinical study.

Another drug, called Aricept, which is used to treat memory problems in Alzheimer's patients, is now being tested on individuals with MS. A recent clinical trial found that Aricept showed improved performance on memory tasks.

Again, it's worth having a conversation with your neurologist about the latest treatments for memory problems, since it's possible that research will make advances in this area soon.

Quick Strategies for Coping with Cognitive Challenges

Fortunately, these marginally effective cognitive drug treatments aren't our only options. Over the years I've learned many cognitive coping strategies from my clients and from MS support group participants. The following practical suggestions have helped thousands improve their ability to deal with cognitive issues. Perhaps they will help you as well.

> Set up some type of organization system that works for you. There are many to choose from. I use a Palm Pilot. But my favorite solution is two huge wall calendars that I hang side-by-side over my desk. I have my husband write in any social appointments that we need to attend together, as well as vacations and days that he will be out of town. I also keep my appointments there so that I can always see at a glance what is coming up. It helps me to pace myself when I can see in advance what the week has in store for me. I use dry-erase markers and reuse the calendars over and over.

> Use sticky-notes as reminders. Keep them in your purse, on your desk, and in your car. Leave them on the front door to remind you of what you have to do that day. Put them on your car dashboard so you don't forget the errands you need to run.

> Program frequently used phone numbers into your phone so that you don't have to remember so many numbers.

> Always keep keys, glasses, watches, and purse, or wallet in the same spot. This reduces panic and frustrating searching time. Whenever possible, maintain a routine.

> Make good use of your computer. Most come with personal information management systems. You can even program many of these to sound an alarm to remind you of appointments or tasks.

> Plan to do your mentally demanding tasks when you normally have the most energy. My husband and close friends know that I can't make important decisions after 7:00 P.M.

Reduce distractions such as music or TV background noise when you're trying to concentrate.

When it's important to remember something or someone, write it down. Always log your debit card entries and check withdrawals as you make them.

Call your home and leave yourself a voice message if you're concerned that you might forget something. It's fun to come home and find a cheerful message from yourself on the machine.

Do one thing at a time. Break projects down into small segments.

Most importantly, talk honestly with your friends and family about the difficulties you may have with your memory. It hurts to be viewed by those you love as lazy or indifferent. You will need to help others understand why you forget things or miss appointments; otherwise, they will assume you are inconsiderate.

Andrea's case is a good example. She came into my office one day on the verge of tears, having just had a huge fight with her husband, Ken. Earlier in the day, Andrea had forgotten to take Cindy, their 12-year-old daughter, to an important follow-up appointment with the dentist. Cindy called her dad, complaining about how her mother was always forgetting everything. Ken called Andrea and yelled, "If I have to do all the chores around the house and go to work, the least you can do is remember to take care of our daughter." Andrea was devastated. Not only did she feel guilty for missing the long-awaited appointment, but her husband's anger and resentment humiliated her. Clearly, everyone in the family was impacted by Andrea's MS-related cognitive problems.

In the past, Ken had been very sympathetic toward Andrea's physical limitations. Although he did get frustrated at times, as all caregivers do, he understood the physical implications of MS and therefore was able to cope with that reality. However, Ken was unaware that cognitive problems can also develop in MS patients. Andrea was afraid to mention her problems because she didn't want to be seen as incompetent or put an additional burden on Ken.

Once Andrea saw that hiding her cognitive difficulties was causing more harm than good, she was able to openly discuss her memory problems. Andrea shared a brochure from the MS society with Ken and Cindy called *Solving Cognitive Problems*, which helped her to explain the effects of cognitive dysfunction in MS patients (see the Resources section for information on obtaining this booklet).

With a bit of education and improved communication, Ken and Andrea began to develop their own system of checks and balances to make sure that important appointments weren't missed.

The Facts about MS Cognitive Dysfunction

As you share your cognitive concerns with your family and friends, it may help to have a few facts at your disposal:

- ❖ Although common, most cognitive difficulties experienced by MS patients are mild.

- ❖ Cognitive problems can occur at any stage of the disease.

- ❖ There is little correlation between how long you've had the disease and the severity of cognitive impairments.

- ❖ Unlike people with Alzheimer's disease, people with MS may stabilize at any time and have no further progression. MS-related cognitive dysfunction is rarely as severe as is seen in Alzheimer's.

- ❖ Just as is the case with physical symptoms, MS patients can't improve their cognitive problems by simply trying harder.

- ❖ Cognitive problems are not a result of an emotional disorder. They are a caused by damage done to the brain by the disease.

These facts can help alleviate concerns your family may have about your cognitive problems and prevent further misunderstanding and confusion about your symptoms.

When cognitive impairments affect your performance at work, you may decide to talk with your boss about the issue. Although every situation is unique, being up-front can often allow you to work around the problems.

For instance, Tony worked in the human resources department of a hospital. He had been living with MS for 10 years, but had only recently noticed changes in his ability to process information and multi-task. He had to ask for things to be repeated and often "spaced out" and forgot important meetings. Naturally, his boss began to notice these problems and he started to criticize Tony for his poor performance. At one point, he even asked Tony if he had a drinking problem. (It is not uncommon for others to make this assumption about people with MS.)

Finally, Tony went to his doctor to get an explanation for the changes he had noticed in himself. After ruling out depression, the doctor concluded that Tony was suffering from MS-related cognitive impairment and he recommended cognitive rehabilitation. Tony was up-front with his boss about what the problem was and what he was doing to address it. His boss, in turn, was relieved to know what was going on and became much more forgiving of Tony's mistakes. He also offered to make adjustments to the work environment to make things easier for Tony. The rehabilitation therapist was able to give Tony several practical suggestions that he was able to apply at work.

Although not every employer will be as accommodating as Tony's, it can ease tension when your supervisor understands that you're fighting MS symptoms and are not simply lazy, apathetic, or abusing alcohol. (You may want to consult an employment attorney before you tell your employer about your illness. Unfortunately, I have heard reports of discrimination resulting from disclosing an MS diagnosis to employers.)

⌘ ⌘ ⌘

In this chapter you've learned how to recognize MS-related cognitive impairments and have also learned several strategies to cope with these symptoms. I encourage you to address these issues so that you might reduce some of the frustration and misunderstandings that these cognitive problems can cause.

Families Speak Out:
Letters from Loved Ones

My wife got the MS diagnosis, but sometimes it feels
like the whole family has it.

— *Pete, husband of an MS patient*

This book wouldn't be complete without a chapter dedicated to
the families of MS patients. When one family member gets MS,
the entire family is ultimately affected. Family members may work
extra hours, do extra chores, and care for us when we can't care for
ourselves. They're often the people who hang in there and go the
extra mile when it's needed. They can be our strength when we
feel weak, our hope when we feel hopeless, and our reason for getting up each day. They worry about us and wish that they could
make us better. Our loved ones are often the unsung heroes in the
MS story.

In these next few pages we will focus on caregivers. Here, they
are given a voice to freely share the pain, challenges, frustrations,
and rewards of loving someone with MS. If you're a caregiver, you
may recognize similarities to your own experiences in their stories.
As an MS patient, you may find that reading the following essays is
painful. My hope is that the emotions shared in this section can

serve as an impetus for patients to talk with loved ones and explore
how family and caregivers feel and what *they* need.

First, we must acknowledge that an MS diagnosis can unex-
pectedly disrupt every aspect of family life. Loved ones are put in
the unimaginably difficult position of not knowing how severe the
disease will become or what will ultimately be required of them as
caregivers. Since MS often strikes early in life, young spouses are
forced to contemplate an uncertain future that is full of responsibilities for which they may not be ready. The vows spoken, "in sick-
ness and in health," are tested much too soon. MS can test the
strongest of marriages and friendships, and yet, the majority of
families do find a way to cope.

In fact, the divorce rate among couples in which one spouse
has MS is no higher than the national average. It stands to reason
that if a marriage is strong to begin with, MS can deepen the commitment that couples share. However, if tension was pervasive in
the relationship before the MS diagnosis, the added burden of the
disease will often prove too much for the marriage to withstand.
This is true of any crisis that a family may encounter. The key to
keeping the relationship healthy and balanced, once again, comes
back to the depth of love and commitment and the quality of communication.

Keep Talking

Oftentimes, family members are frustrated by their inability to express how the disease makes *them* feel—in some ways like the frustration MS patients feel. Loved ones are ashamed to admit that
they experience normal frustrations, concerns, and doubts. "How
can I say anything about how hard this is for me when she's the one
who suffers with this disease? She never escapes from it," says
Howard, the husband and caregiver of an MS patient for seven
years. Frequently, caregivers feel selfish or guilty for sharing their
honest feelings about MS. They may be afraid that if they speak
openly about how difficult the disease is for them, it will hurt or
upset the person with MS. Tragically, this silence creates a huge

chasm that many couples never bridge, and, inevitably, resentment results. Since it's so difficult and yet so important for loved ones to share how they feel about the impact MS has on their lives, it may be up to the patient to start this conversation. The exercise provided in Chapter 2, "MS Diagnosis Questionnaire," is a good way to start this dialogue.

Many Voices, Many Views

After speaking with many different family members and friends of MS patients about how the disease has impacted their lives, I've selected the following shared experiences to show the different ways that others perceive and respond to MS. Their responses vary as widely as do the patients' symptoms and experiences.

WHEN A SPOUSE/PARTNER HAS MS

Caregiving responsibilities can be as varied as MS symptoms, which is why a wide range of responses are considered in this chapter. After reading the uncensored thoughts and feelings on how the disease impacts others, you may be relieved to learn that you're not alone in your conflicted feelings about loving someone with a chronic illness.

When loved ones answer the question, "How does MS impact *your* life?" a wide range of feelings may surface: Guilt, anger, frustration, sadness, helplessness, empathy, hopelessness, fear, disappointment, and the desire to escape are often mentioned. All of these feelings are valid and understandable. Your response will be unique to you, your relationship, and your situation. The following are just a few perspectives on how it can feel to be a caregiver:

Jim, 38, husband of an MS patient since 1999

When my wife was first diagnosed with MS, we were both young. At first we thought it was a death sentence. Neither of us knew much about the disease. Over the years we've learned how to deal with it better. The biggest challenge for me is that we both used to be extremely active. My wife's love of hiking and skiing and boating were all things that attracted me to her. But now, she's able to do less and less. If she feels up to taking a short walk with me, it's a big deal. Anything we do has to be well planned. The spontaneity has disappeared from our lives.

To look at us and our life together, things seem normal. This is one of the reasons it's so hard to explain to people how our life has changed. No, she's not in a wheelchair and she can still do what she needs to do, but not what she wants to do. We're still young; we're supposed to slow down in our eighties, not our thirties. If it's like this now, what's it going to be like down the road? Just reading this makes me feel guilty for complaining because she hasn't gotten much worse. I love my wife and I'm going to stick by her no matter what happens. I see how strong she is and what she endures and I know that my annoyances don't compare to her daily battles, but I still have these thoughts and I feel really frustrated.

Jim expresses what many spouses feel. He's disappointed because his fantasy of what life was supposed to be like with his young wife has been altered. It's terribly difficult to accept that our lives are limited by disease. He must not only learn to adapt to these new circumstances, but he's trying to brace himself for the future by anticipating the possibility that his wife could become further disabled. Jim also speaks of guilt for having these feelings.

However, just as with patients, anxiety is reduced when family members focus on how well their loved one is doing today and deal with the present reality. Also, since MS is a marathon, not a sprint, it's important for Jim to find ways to continue doing the activities he loves. He still has many years left to pursue his passions. Finding a group of buddies who enjoy hiking or skiing or biking may be an appropriate compromise since his wife can no longer join him. If Jim can find an outlet for his adventurous side, then he may feel less frustrated by his wife's limitations and, in turn, be able to appreciate the short walks that they're still able to take together.

Many caregivers stuff their feelings because they compare their pain to that of their loved one. But each of us suffers in our own way when chronic illness strikes a family. Emotional pain can't be measured or compared; it just is. MS exacts sacrifice from everyone who is touched by it, not just from the patient. All feelings are valid and must be honored, or distance will inevitably occur between loved ones.

The helplessness that family members feel when they have a loved one who suffers from MS can be demoralizing. Caregivers want nothing more than to take away the pain and disability MS causes, and yet they're constantly aware that nothing can be done to reverse the diagnosis. This defenselessness periodically creates feelings of failure, depression, and guilt.

Lenny, husband of an MS patient since 1994

Clearly, MS has changed my wife's life. While not quite so dramatic, it has also affected my life, as well as our life as a couple. The disease has created tension that frequently arises from me trying to live my life to the fullest while having to constantly throttle back to accommodate my wife, whose MS-induced fatigue cuts short most activities that don't involve resting. I'm angry at the disease—not the patient—for a certain loss of freedom and of the carefree approach to life that I—and we—once had. It has curtailed our social life and forced me to spend more time alone, since my wife can't fully engage in all the social and physical activities that we've enjoyed in the past. Everything we do requires advance planning so that my wife doesn't get too tired, too hungry, too hot, or too cold. It doesn't sound like that big of a deal, but her environment each day has to be as controlled as possible to keep her symptoms at bay. We both have to work hard to find things we can still enjoy doing together.

It took me years to really understand my wife's symptoms, especially her truck-stopping fatigue. It has also been a challenge to give her all the support she needs without getting on her nerves. I constantly ask her how she feels in order to gauge her well-being. My biggest concern is that I'm not doing enough for her to make her life easier.

Perhaps the greatest impact this disease has had on us was our decision not to have children. We were planning to have a child when my wife was diagnosed. We decided to see how she reacted to the medication. After a year, she felt having a child would be too much for her. This was a blow to me because I had always wanted to have one or two kids. I wanted kids before I even wanted a wife. Of course, I didn't want her health to suffer unless she wanted nothing more than to have children. But she didn't. So we didn't. Both of us would have made great parents. MS robbed me of the opportunity to be a father and to have a family.

On the bright side, MS forced my wife to tone down her A-type personality as it relates to work. She can no longer work a full-time job, which, before MS, was full-time plus evenings and weekends. Her constant work drove me nuts. She also appreciates nature more, which is one of my passions.

Living with my wife and her MS is frustrating, wonderful, annoying, lovely, and disappointing. In short, I wouldn't trade her no matter what disease she has, or may have in the future. It isn't her fault she contracted this disabling illness. I feel sorry for her and find it a crying shame that someone who once had so much energy, and who still has a zest for life, has to deal with this. Mainly, I feel helpless because I can't do anything to help cure her.

Until a cure is found, there is little you can do to stop MS, but caregivers do make the disease more tolerable and greatly improve the quality of a patient's life. The love, physical support, and emotional sustenance offered to MS patients are what carries them through the day-to-day challenges of this disease. You make a huge difference in your loved one's life with each small act of kindness and care that you provide. These are the meaningful rewards of caregiving.

Lenny also mentions the losses he experiences: the loss of the opportunity for fatherhood and the loss of a more socially and physically active life. Regrettably, caregivers must bear their own losses as well as the losses of the patient. These losses need to be grieved and acknowledged by the family.

Despite all the sorrow this disease has caused, it is interesting to note that Lenny wouldn't trade his wife in for a healthier version. On the contrary, he has a deep desire to support his wife and feels frustrated that he can't do more for her.

Susan, 45, wife of a recently diagnosed MS patient

MS hit us suddenly. My husband had serious vision problems—pain in his eye—then he became unsteady on his feet and was dizzy all the time. After we got the MS diagnosis, things continued to get worse. He has progressive-relapsing MS, which isn't the best kind.

We have a daughter in elementary school and I'm working full-time as a secretary. My husband had to quit his job as an accountant and he's on disability now. He's able to help some with the house chores, but I feel like the entire burden of our family is on my shoulders. He was always the strong one and now he just can't manage most things. Since he became ill he goes to counseling for depression and his doctor put him on antidepressants, but I think I'm the one who needs them. When I imagine him in a wheelchair . . . I just don't know if I can handle it.

I understand that he's the one who's sick and I feel awful about it, but sometimes I think he got off easy. He gets to stay home and he knows that I'll take care of everything. Who's taking care of me? Our daughter still comes to me for everything, but I don't have the time for her. I don't think she knows how to connect with her dad, and now that he's sick, she seems afraid to approach him. At this rate I don't know how I'll go on, but what choice do I have?

Naturally, Susan is feeling overwhelmed by suddenly assuming the entire responsibility for her family. As often happens when someone gets a serious illness, designated roles have changed and in this case, quickly. Not having time to gradually adapt to her husband's disability has caught Susan off guard. She is operating in survival mode and hasn't had time to consider her options. Furthermore, she feels trapped, knowing she can't keep doing it all for everyone, but feeling that she must.

When disability is severe, it's often necessary to seek outside assistance. Unfortunately, many caregivers have a difficult time reaching out and asking for help. They feel as if they're failing when they need others to share the workload. However, when caregivers don't accept help from others, they often end up burning out or becoming sick themselves. Often, family or friends can pitch in. You never know, they may just be waiting for you to ask. Neighbors might be willing to run errands or to watch children. Sometimes you *need* to hire professionals. Church groups, hospital social workers, your doctor's office, or the MS Society may be good resources to help you find the right person.

It's also important to make sure that as a caregiver you don't just assume that you have to do everything. Explore what your spouse may be able to contribute, despite their illness. They may not be able to do things the way they once did, but by getting creative you could discover new ways of getting things done. For example, Susan's husband might be able to do laundry or help prepare food for dinner, even if these tasks were previously her responsibilities. Furthermore, although children should never be the primary caregivers, you may need to ask them to take on additional house chores.

Because caregiving can bring about many strong emotions, such as frustration, loneliness, and resentment, seeking emotional support from outside sources is critical. Attend a caregiver support group or seek family and/or individual therapy. Be sure to make time to go out with friends, or have them over for coffee. Even if you confide in just one friend, you will feel less alone.

Of course, it can be difficult to make time to get away or leave the house when you're providing care for someone, but now there are many excellent Internet caregiver support websites that you can access from a home computer (see the Resources section). It's imperative that the needs of the caregiver are met in order for the relationship to stay healthy. When you don't replenish yourself by using outside sources, your ability to give and provide care will eventually give out.

Stewart, husband of an MS patient since 2004

As challenges appear, I've always been one to view them as an opportunity to experience feelings and to learn.

In the summer of 2004, my wife obtained her credentials as a special education teacher. Her focus was serving the needs of severely disabled children with autism. She loved the opportunity it gave her to focus on a small group of children and found wonderful satisfaction in seeing her students' progress.

As the school year drew to a close, my wife began having difficulties. Her reactions slowed and she had difficulty concentrating. In June she had two back-to-back minor auto accidents that were suspiciously similar—something I felt was caused by more than simple inattentive behavior. I insisted that we see a doctor. In July 2004, after an MRI scan and a spinal tap, the neurologist diagnosed her condition as primary-progressive multiple sclerosis. To say that this diagnosis hit both of us like a "ton of bricks" would be an understatement. The neurologist asked that we return in a week to discuss treatment options.

I spent that week focused on the Internet and its available resources, learning as much as I could about potential treatment options and the nature of this disease. What I uncovered wasn't what I wanted to read. I learned that the drugs utilized to help those with the remitting-relapsing form of this disease have proven ineffective in dealing with patients with PPMS. So it came as no surprise when we met with the neurologist and he recommended we focus on reducing disease symptoms rather than a cure. For us, this meant utilizing medication to help my wife deal with chronic pain. We also learned that she would lose her driver's license for neurological reasons.

In August, my wife started having difficulties walking and we bought a cane. We made a big deal of shopping for one that made an appropriate fashion statement. Later that same month, her fatigue reached a level where she could no longer make the short walk to our local grocery store. Internet shopping came to the rescue. Then I found and purchased a small electric mobility scooter that she could use to make this trip. Since August her condition has continued to progress and we're making accommodations to meet her needs.

With over 20 years in Alcoholics Anonymous, open sharing of my feelings is second nature. When we learned of the diagnosis, I immediately increased the number of my AA meetings. In the many years as an AA participant, I've watched other members utilize the tools of the fellowship in dealing with absolutely horrific situations that most of us would find impossible to cope with. I also knew that AA was not the single solution, and I believed it necessary to seek professional counseling to deal with the emotional aspects of what was going on. Fortunately, through an employee assistance program, counseling services were readily available.

I also chose to share openly with my colleagues at the college where I teach, and with my students, the difficulties we were facing. I wanted people to recognize that if my teaching performance seemed to slip, there was an underlying cause.

In dealing with the daily aspects of this disease, I'm committed to providing whatever my wife needs. Nevertheless, I recognize that my needs are also important. I've adjusted my teaching schedule so that I can be at home to provide caretaker services. I've also taken steps to determine when it would be appropriate to recognize that I can't handle these responsibilities all by myself. Fortunately, I've worked closely with our college nursing faculty in the past on efforts to obtain grants. With our local RN, LVN, and CNA programs in place, when the need arises for us to hire caretaker services, I have a nursing faculty ready to assist me in finding the right caretakers.

If there is a key to my handling of the situation, it's aggressively seeking the advice and help of others. As much as I hate this disease and the terrible things it's doing to my wife, I remain committed not to abandon an approach that will insure a quality lifestyle for her. I am further committed to seek help so that I avoid potential resentments during this passage. Acceptance of the situation and a "one day at a time" approach appears to be serving me well.

Stewart has taken several proactive steps to avoid burnout, and he has developed a long-term care plan to reduce anxiety. Like Stewart, most caregivers, as well as MS patients, agree that support groups are an essential outlet for their feelings and a source of great comfort when they're overwhelmed. Stewart was fortunate enough to have an existing support group established through his participation in Alcoholics Anonymous meetings. A support group doesn't necessarily have to be a formal caregivers meeting. Your support might come from your weekly golf game, your church, or your book club.

Richard, husband of an MS patient since 1990

I'm a father of three kids, ages 18, 16, and 10. My wife was diagnosed with MS in 1991. She's still able to work, and she doesn't want to quit and have to accept being labeled disabled at 36.

She's my high-school sweetheart, and we've been together 20-plus years. She recently passed from remissive to progressive MS, and they started her on more medications, which her make her feel lousy.

Slowly, over the years, I've shouldered more and more of the household load. Now I also find myself attending things without her, like the kids' sports, my sports, evenings out with friends, just about all things social. I'm 38 and starting to get stress-related illness. I'm so drained that I can't see the light at the end of the tunnel. I hate MS like I never hated anything else, and I resent what its turning me into. For the first time, I have serious doubts of making it through. Sorry for venting like this. . . . I'm afraid of being judged!

Sometimes caregivers do feel like throwing in the towel. But before any reactive decisions are made, it's important to determine if you no longer love your partner, or if the burden of caregiving has simply become too much. These are two entirely separate issues. Richard has gone through a great deal with his wife and has remained with her so far, so something is keeping him in the marriage. It's clear that Richard hates the disease, not his wife. This is a critical distinction. The burden of doing all the household chores and the loneliness of attending most social events alone are two issues that can be addressed. Richard will feel less resentful and his wife might have more energy to participate in some of the fun activities that are going on outside the home if they seek some outside assistance for housekeeping. Given the age of their children, it's also reasonable to ask the kids to pitch in around the house. Setting aside time each week to discuss how the family will divide household tasks might be a good way to start getting the kids more involved in helping out.

Most importantly, Richard and his wife need to carve out time and begin talking to each other about how MS is impacting their lives. Perhaps, if they can afford it, Richard's wife could cut back her hours at work. This could give her more time and energy to help out with the house and join in family outings. If she understands how seriously the disease is impacting her marriage, she may be willing to make these changes in order to give Richard some relief. By hiding his feelings from her, Richard doesn't give his wife a chance to address his concerns and potentially take the steps necessary to save the marriage.

A red flag pops up when Richard mentions that he has developed "stress-related" illnesses. As a caregiver, it's crucial that you maintain your own health. This includes going to see your doctor on a regular basis, getting exercise, eating right, taking your own prescribed medications, and finding a positive way to release your emotions. Too often, caregivers become so involved in the care of their loved one that they neglect their own physical needs and then their own health suffers. When this happens, families can collapse into crisis.

WHEN A FRIEND HAS MS

The effects of MS can be very confusing for friends and difficult for them to understand. When an MS patient's energy is limited, they may have to slow down and socialize less. Oftentimes patients have to cancel plans or go home early, and this can feel like rejection to friends. Those who suffer from cognitive impairments may forget confidences shared by friends or may seem disinterested in the concerns of their friends. The friendship can begin to require a great deal of tolerance and patience. But what true friendship doesn't?

Rose, 38, best friend of an MS patient since 1998

When I watch what this disease does to my friend, it makes me so angry. Sometimes it seems like it's stealing her essence.

She only has about three or four hours of quality time in the day. It literally takes away her life and forces her to dole out her time and emotions very carefully. I find myself holding back and not always being honest with her because I don't want to cause an attack to kick in. I used to just let it all out with her, and that was what made our relationship so special, but now I'm careful because she seems more fragile.

On the positive side, I feel closer to her because I'm really learning what it's like for her to live with this disease day-in and day-out. She shares her fears, concerns, sadness, and anger—and that has added a new, deeper dimension to our friendship. She's let me in to see her vulnerable side and her pain and I don't know if that would have happened if she hadn't gotten sick.

When these things happen, try to consider that having a friend with MS can also teach you about coping with the unexpected. They can inspire and support you to overcome your own obstacles. As Rose mentions, if both of you are willing, you can connect on a deeper level and develop a more meaningful relationship as you navigate the rough waters of chronic illness together.

WHEN A PARENT HAS MS

Most of our rewarding relationships demand more from us than we ever knew we could give.

Lucy, 16, daughter of a recently diagnosed MS patient

I try to help out around the house and have a good attitude, but sometimes I feel really pissed about it. Other kids are going out, meeting at Starbucks or down at the school field, and I'm stuck having to clean and cook and do the stuff my mom used to do. When I see how bad she feels, it makes me feel awful, but still, I've lost my temper and told her that I hated her for getting sick. What kind of person am I? Nobody at school understands. I can't really talk with my friends about it. I'm afraid that they'll think my family is weird.

Regardless of their age, most caregivers feel tremendous anger at one time or another. This anger can easily be directed toward the person who is ill. Tempers flare, words are spoken that can't be taken back, and feelings are hurt. Fortunately, these outbursts are usually temporary and result from feelings of extreme frustration, disappointment, and perhaps fatigue.

When a teen like Lucy is helping to care for a parent with MS, their grades may suffer, or they may be tempted to turn to drugs or alcohol as an escape from the difficult realities of a life that seems unfair.

Just like adults, young caregivers must find a positive outlet for the inevitable painful feelings that arise when caring for a loved one who is ill. When feelings of anger are dealt with early on—before they reach a boiling point—conflicts can be minimized.

Kids should be encouraged to develop a relationship with an adult in whom they can confide and express all their feelings without the guilt and remorse that comes from blasting the ill parent. Ministers, counselors, other family members, and MS support groups for kids are all possible resources that can provide support and understanding.

Tammy, 21, father diagnosed with MS in 2004

My father was diagnosed with MS about a year ago. I will turn 22 soon and my father is 48.

This year I spent my father's birthday in the hospital with him. The last year has been really hard. Just when I thought I was getting a grip on life after moving to another state and getting a steady job that I loved and my own apartment, this happened. I've gone through a lot of shock, frustration, anger, more frustration, depression, and various other feelings—things that I assume come along with coping with a parent's incurable disease. I'm tired of the pity in people's eyes when I tell them my father is sick. I'm tired of horrible people thinking my father is a drunken bum on the street when he stumbles. I hate it that I feel that my role as a child has been reversed and that I'm now the one that has to keep an eye on my dad and fight the fight for him against others' opinions.

How do I cope with this? How do you handle the nerve-racking thought that any day another attack might come?

How? How do I fight this fight alone? I don't have anyone to support me. My father is all that I have.

I used to tell people all the time, should anything happen to my father, my world would fall apart. And it has.

Tammy's young life has been flipped upside down. Just when she was venturing out into the world to create a life of her own, her father suddenly needed her care. At the time she wrote this, Tammy was facing conflicting feelings about the role-reversal that she was being thrust into. It's frightening to see the person you've always counted on and relied upon become dependent, and it's natural for Tammy to feel discouraged.

Although Tammy went through a range of emotions, loneliness seemed to be the most troubling for her. Since she had no family support, Tammy had no immediate person to turn to for advice and comfort.

Tammy eventually found some answers on how to cope with her isolation through the Internet. She discovered a chat room that is specifically designed to help MS caregivers. This has become a survival tool for her. Not only does it provide emotional support, but she's getting practical advice about caregiving options and other resources that are available to her.

Tammy also learned that she could still count on her father for the emotional support he had always provided her. Once she told him how she felt, they were able to share their sadness and comfort each other. Just because her dad has MS doesn't mean he can't still be there for her.

WHEN A CHILD HAS MS

Dorothy, mother of an MS patient since 1996

One day I got a call from my 28-year-old daughter, and she told me her doctor had tested her and confirmed she had MS. I felt like the end of the world had come. My first inclination was to fly out to see her but she told me that she and her husband were coping and doing fine. I decided to let the newlyweds work through this together and not interfere. This is a decision

I've always regretted. It was tough to sit at home and think that my beautiful, creative, energetic daughter had been given a life sentence of MS. As I've learned more about the treatments available, I've changed my feelings about that, but I still worry that she will end up blind or in a wheelchair. My husband and I have changed our will to help pay for any future health-care expenses she may incur, and we've built a home that is handicapped accessible and fully paid for, should she ever need it.

We cope by praying and sharing our feelings together. Our family finds that love and optimism and being proactive can really help the situation. We try to focus on the things we can do to help.

Most parents want to protect and take care of their adult children with MS just at the time when the patient is struggling to become self-sufficient or start their own separate life. This can create tension and conflict as families try to determine what is considered helpful and what is interfering.

In Dorothy's case, she has made the constructive decision to focus on what she can do for her daughter without being intrusive. Looking toward the future, Dorothy has made an effort to help take care of her daughter financially. This is something within Dorothy's power and it gives the entire family a sense of comfort and greater security.

Taking Care of You

After reading these letters, you may be struck by the great many similarities between how MS impacts both caregivers and patients. The coping strategies for stress, anger, grief, communication, loneliness, and depression suggested in this book can be applied to anyone whose life is disrupted by chronic illness, and I encourage both caregivers and patients to use these tools.

Finally, it's widely believed that the key to avoiding burnout as a caregiver is to keep your life in balance. Naturally, when someone is sick, most of the care and attention is directed toward them. The patient is given the support of her doctor, her medical team, concerned friends and loved ones, but often the caregiver can feel left alone in the shadows. If this is your experience, it will be up to you to get your needs met.

A few suggestions that might make caregiving easier include the following:

- ❖ Do things for yourself as well as others.

- ❖ Maintain your outside interests and friendships.

- ❖ Find people who can give you a break when you need it.

- ❖ Set up your home to allow the patient to be as independent as possible and reduce their dependence on you.

- ❖ Arrange your home environment so it is safe for your loved one to move around and to maximize their mobility. Remove rugs and cords that can be tripped on. If the patient is confined to a wheelchair, make your home as handicapped accessible as possible. If you can afford it, add ramps and renovate your home so that the kitchen and bath are accessible.

- ❖ Ask the doctor for an occupational therapy referral. These folks are skilled at doing home assessments and in suggesting ways to reduce physical strain on both the patient and the caregiver.

- ❖ Have the patient wear a lifeline device that would allow them to call for help if you were gone from the home and they were to fall.

- ❖ Create a list of people you can count on to help you if you are feeling burned out. Post it by the phone and use it before you reach the end of your rope.

- ❖ Depending on how much care the patient needs, you might want to consider adult day care or hiring an aid to come in during the day.

- ❖ Work with the patient to determine chores or responsibilities they might be able to handle on their own.

❖ Get training on the most efficient approaches to transferring, bathing, giving injections, toileting, and dressing techniques if you are providing this level of care. You can get a home health referral from the doctor, and, in addition to providing training, they may also be able to relieve you from some of these responsibilities.

❖ When friends offer to help, accept their help, and be specific about what tasks they might take on for you.

❖ Attend caregiver support groups (see the Resources section) and maintain a social life outside of caregiving activities.

Taking care of yourself isn't selfish. It's a necessity if you're going to go the distance as a caregiver. It's often said, "You can't take care of anyone else if you don't take care of yourself first." This is a statement to take to heart.

chapter
fourteen

Ending on a
Positive Note

Although everyone experiences this disease differently, MS demands bravery from us all. It requires us to look for good in bad situations. It forces us to grow up and as Dr. Phil says, "Get real." Often it tests our limits, and we must dig down deep to come up with enough strength just to get through the day. Each loss, each challenge, each obstacle can either break us or make us stronger. MS patients are tough birds. Those whom I've met are resilient. In fact, they are some of the mightiest, funniest, kindest, and most inspiring people I could ever hope to know. The majority of MS patients I talk with, regardless of how severe their disability is, are fighters who refuse to be defined by their illness. I'll admit, the MS club is not a group I would have ever asked to join, but when I think of all the incredible people I have come to know since being diagnosed twelve years ago, I'm certain that my life is vastly richer than before I had the disease.

What I've learned from others who have this disease is that although MS takes away a great deal, it can give us gifts as well, depending on how you look at it. I've seen MS bring out the best in people. It can teach us to be patient, to be kind, to be aware, to love deeply, and to live intensely. It can show us how to truly open our hearts and let those who love us take care of us. It can help us appreciate the simple moments that most people take for granted. It boils life down to its very essence and reveals what is true—that we should make each day on this earth count. Fortunately, every day we are given that choice. My hope is that this book will make that choice easier for you.

Hope for the Future

⌘ ⌘ ⌘

An Afterword
by Dr. Stanley Cohan

The past 10 years have been challenging and rewarding for many people with MS. For the first time, therapeutic agents that significantly reduce clinical relapses and the progression of physical disability have become available. However, there are major deficiencies in currently available therapeutic regimens. These include a lack of sustained control of disease activity for many patients, with only modest reduction in relapse risk, and/or progression of their physical disability. Side effects of medications, in many cases, have significant negative impact on quality of life. There also continue to be difficulties in reliably establishing the diagnosis of MS in many patients, despite the enormous beneficial impact of the MRI scanning, which Allison mentioned earlier, in improving diagnostic sensitivity and accuracy.

What should our future goals be?

1. Clearly, more sensitive and more specific diagnostic tools are needed to facilitate earlier and more accurate diagnoses, particularly since early initiation of therapy is likely to improve patient prognosis in many cases.

2. New therapies that are superior in controlling MS, and that are safe and well tolerated, are needed.

3. New therapeutic strategies should aim to prevent MS from developing at all, pointing to the need for diagnostic tools

that can reliably predict who is going to develop MS before it becomes clinically manifest.

4. In patients who already have MS, therapy must better aim to control the biological processes by which injury to the nervous system occurs, and to repair damaged myelin, nerve fibers, and nerve cells.

Treatment Now and in the Future

Once MS is established in a person, attention must focus on medications that reduce, or preferably, turn off the disease. It is widely acknowledged that the MS disease process is driven by the immune system, which becomes misdirected and inappropriately attacks the nervous system, damaging or destroying myelin, nerve fibers, and nerve cells.

Early attempts to control this inappropriate, self-destructive immune system dysfunction employed drugs that are very robust depressors of immune function, usually cancer chemotherapeutic agents and corticosteroids. These medications are still used in many patients. However, unacceptable toxicity in many cases and lack of sustained benefit in controlling disease activity are major shortcomings of these medications. In addition, these medications are nonspecific and may suppress immune function totally rather than suppressing just the portion of the immune system attacking the nervous system. This may leave patients more vulnerable to serious infections and reduce their ability to destroy tumor cells.

Newer medications, the beta-interferons and glatarimer, alter the immune system in ways that reduce nervous system damage, but do not suppress the immune system's ability to fight infections or suppress the growth of cancer cells. But as noted above, these agents can produce adverse side effects, provide only modest control of MS in many patients, and provide little or no benefit for people with non-relapsing, progressive forms of MS.

A new generation of medications is being developed that is more specific, in that the medications selectively alter the behavior of the immune system's white blood cells that are directed against the nervous system, while sparing the protective role of the immune system for the rest of the body. One of these new medications selectively blocks white blood cells entering the brain, while other new agents seek to alter the inappropriate, self-destructive behavior of the immune system (called autoimmunity), while sparing normal immune function. Autoimmunity is probably genetically determined, and as noted above, once identified, these genes may be turned off and prevent destructive autoimmune activity.

Why do white blood cells "know" to travel to the nervous system and to specific sites within the nervous system? The nervous system sends out chemical signals (called chemokines) that attract specific types of white blood cells to specific sites within the nervous system. Blocking or inhibiting these chemokines is another potentially important therapeutic opportunity, which could result in preventing the immune system from attacking the nervous system, because it would be unable to "find" the nervous system.

WHAT ABOUT NERVOUS SYSTEM REPAIR?

There are three strategies for nervous system repair:

1. Stimulate inherent repair mechanisms of damaged, but not destroyed, nerves by using therapeutic agents that activate nerve-building or nerve-repair genes, or that mimic the proteins these genes produce. We know that such genes exist.

2. For nerves that have survived an immune attack but are dying, or are destined to die prematurely, we should be able to block the biochemical steps leading to cell death by shutting off the "suicide" genes, some of which have already been identified. Important progress has been made in this area, but no therapeutic agents have as yet been developed.

3. The death of nerve cells and loss of nerve fibers appears to be the most important cause of major functional impair-

ment and the progression of permanent disability. It is the replacement of lost nervous system tissue which stem cell research is attempting to address. The hope is to cure disability by regenerating new, healthy nervous tissue. Stem cell transplantation has been used therapeutically in a small number of MS patients, but it is premature to draw any conclusions as to the potential success of this approach, or as to whether stem cell techniques currently employed will be replaced by better techniques and/or better stem cell lines.

WHAT ABOUT TREATING MS SYMPTOMS?

For many, if not all MS patients, symptoms resulting from nervous system damage are major factors affecting their functional status and quality of life. Left untreated, these symptoms can reduce quality of life, even if the MS disease process is under control. All these symptoms are important and they should be treated if they have an adverse impact on the patient. These symptoms include excessive fatigue, increasing cognitive difficulties (particularly memory, concentration, multi-tasking, and speed of thinking), depression, anxiety, weakness, pain and other sensory disturbances, spasticity, urinary bladder dysfunction, impaired sexual function, and infections.

Many of these issues have been discussed in detail previously in this book. Suffice it to say, these problems should not be ignored, glossed-over, or treated half-heartedly by your physicians or nurses. If you are not being asked about these symptoms or you are not receiving vigorous therapy for them, it is extremely important that you become a vocal and persistent advocate for treatment of these disease symptoms. It can spell the difference between a successful and unsuccessful outcome.

THE FUTURE LOOKS PROMISING

The future for patients with MS is exciting and should be viewed with optimism. There are currently so many types of therapeutic opportunities, and the number and types of therapeutic strategies will only further expand with the passage of time. Critical insights pertaining to the causes and mechanisms of the disease, combined with new technologies, offer realistic hope for cures for MS. Improved insights and technologies will not only result in better diagnostic accuracy, but could eventually lead to diagnostic screening tests that can reliably identify a person at risk before they develop MS, before they develop symptoms or abnormalities on MRI scans, and lead to medical interventions that prevent MS from developing. Clinical medicine anticipates the development of blood tests to track disease activity, so we can determine how well medication is working, rather than waiting until new injury in the form of MRI changes or new symptoms informs us that a change in medication is required.

This exciting future is not just wishful thinking. We already have the insights and technology needed to achieve many of these goals. Thus, it is essential that every MS patient does everything possible to preserve their physical and emotional health so that they may be in a position to experience the maximum benefits that each new improvement in MS care brings.

Suggested Reading

⌘ ⌘ ⌘

Barrett M. *Sexuality and Multiple Sclerosis.* 3rd ed. Toronto: Multiple Sclerosis Society of Canada, 1991.

Blackstone, Margaret. *The First Year: Multiple Sclerosis.* New York: Marlowe & Company, 2003.

Branden, Nathaniel. *The Six Pillars of Self-Esteem.* New York: Bantam Books, 1994.

Burns, David D. *Feeling Good: The New Mood Therapy.* New York: Avon Books, 1980.

Corn, Laura. *101 Nights of Grrreat Sex: Secret Sealed Seductions for Fun Loving Couples.* New York: Park Avenue Publishers, 2000.

Cox, Darcy, and Laura Julian. "Cognitive Dysfunction in Multiple Sclerosis." In *Multiple Sclerosis: Etiology, Diagnosis and New Treatment Strategies* (Current Clinical Neurology), edited by Michael, J. Olek, 91–102. Totowa, New Jersey: Humana Press Inc., 2004.

Cooper, Laura D. *Insurance Solutions—Plan Well, Live Better: A Workbook for People with a Chronic Disease or Disability.* New York: Demos Medical Publishing, 2001.

Didion, Joan. *The Year of Magical Thinking.* New York: Knopf, 2005.

Gray, John. *Men Are from Mars, Women Are from Venus.* New York: HarperCollins Publishers, 1992.

Holland, Nancy J., T. Jock Murray, and Stephen C. Reingold. *Multiple Sclerosis: A Guide for the Newly Diagnosed.* 2nd ed. New York: Demos Medical Publishing, 2002.

Kabat-Zinn, Jon. *Full Catastrophe Living.* New York: Dell Publishing, 1990.

Kalb, Rosalind C. *Multiple Sclerosis: A Guide for Families.* New York: Demos Medical Publishing, 1998.

Kenyon, Jane. *Constance.* St. Paul, MN: Graywolf Press, 1993.

Krupp, Lauren B. *Fatigue in Multiple Sclerosis*. New York: Demos Medical Publishing, 2004.

Larson, Andrew, and Ivy Ingram Larson. *The Gold Coast Cure*. Deerfield Beach, FL: Health Communications Inc., 2005.

Lerner, Harriet. *The Dance of Anger*. New York: HarperCollins Publishers, Inc., 1997.

Lombardo, Gerald, and Henry Ehrlich. *Sleep to Save Your Life: The Complete Guide to Living Longer and Healthier Through Restorative Sleep*. New York: HarperCollins, 2005.

Lustbader, Wendy. *Counting on Kindness*. New York: Free Press, 1991.

Maas, James B., Megan L Wherry, David J. Axelrod, Barbara R. Hogan, and Jennifer Bloomin. *Power Sleep: The Revolutionary Program That Prepares Your Mind for Peak Performance*. New York: HarperCollins, 1998.

May, Rollo. *Man's Search for Himself*. New York: Dell Publishing, 1967.

McCue, Kathleen, and Ron Bonn. *How to Help Children Through a Parents' Serious Illness*. New York: St. Martin's Press, 1994.

McKay, Mathew, and Patrick Fanning. *Self-Esteem*. New York: St. Martin's Press, 1987.

Miller, Alice. *Brandished Knowledge: Facing Childhood Injuries*. New York: Anchor Books, 1990.

Naparstek, Belleruth. *Staying Well with Guided Imagery*. New York: Warner Books, Inc., 1995.

Nichols, Judith Lynn, and Her Online Group of MS Sisters. *Women Living with Multiple Sclerosis*. Alameda, CA: Hunter House, 1999.

Nichols, Judith Lynn, and Her Online Group of MS Sisters. *Living Beyond Multiple Sclerosis*. Alameda, CA: Hunter House, 2000.

O'Connor, Paul. *Multiple Sclerosis: The Facts You Need*. Toronto, Ontario: Key Porter Books, 2002.

Pert, Candace. *Molecules of Emotion*. New York: Touchstone, 1997.

Remen, Rachel Naomi. *Kitchen Table Wisdom*. New York: Riverhead Books, 1996.

Rogers, Carl. *On Becoming a Person*. New York: Constable & Robinson, Ltd. 2004.

Rosner, Louis J., and Shelley Ross. *Multiple Sclerosis*. New York: Fireside, 1992.

Sarton, May. *Journal of Solitude*. New York: W.W. Norton & Company, Inc., 1973.

Schwiebert, Pat. *Symptoms of Grief*. 2003. http://www.griefwatch.com/ (4 Jan. 2006).

Solomon, Andrew. *The Noonday Demon*. New York: Simon and Schuster, 2001.

Tannen, Deborah. *You Just Don't Understand*. New York: Harper-Collins, 1990.

Viorst, Judith. *Necessary Losses*. New York: Fawcett Gold Medal, 1986.

Waldman, Jackie. *People with MS and the Courage to Give*. York Beach, ME: Red Wheel/Weiser LLC, 2003.

Weil, Andrew. *Spontaneous Healing*. New York: Alfred A. Knopf, Inc., 1995.

Williams, Montel. *Climbing Higher*. New York: New American Library, 2005.

Resources

⌘ ⌘ ⌘

General Information and Referrals

Accent on Information
P.O. Box 700
Bloomington, IL 61702   (304) 378-2961
A computerized system of information to help the disabled deal with
activities of daily living and home-care issues. A small fee is charged,
but services will not be denied to those who can't pay.

Consortium of Multiple Sclerosis Centers
c/o Gimbel MS Center at Holy Name Hospital
718 Teaneck Rd.
Teaneck NJ 07666   (201) 837-0727
Website: www.info.mscare.org

Disability Resource Center (jjMarketing)
1205 Savoy St., Suite 101
San Diego CA 92107   (800) 787-8444
Website: www.blvd.com
A directory of products and services.

Equal Employment Opportunity Commission
1801 L St. NW, 10th Fl.
Washington DC 20507   (800) 669-4000
Website: www.eeoc.gov

National Council on Disability
1331 F Street NW, Suite 850
Washington DC 20004   (202) 272-2004
Website: www.ncd.gov

National Multiple Sclerosis Society
733 3rd Ave.
New York NY 10017-3288   (800) 344-4867
Website: www.nationalmssociety.org

Sears Home Health Care Catalog
P.O. Box 3123
Naperville IL 60566   (800) 326-1750
Includes medical equipment products and adaptive clothing.

Social Security Administration
6401 Security Blvd.
Baltimore MD 21235   (800) 772-1213
Call to apply for Social Security benefits.

Meditation

Full Catastrophe Living, by Jon Kabat-Zinn. This is a great book for
the meditation novice. It comes with several exercises and illustrates
in simple language the benefits of meditation practice. It also provides
excellent information on breathing exercises, yoga, and relaxation. It
can be purchased through Amazon.com.

You can also order the *Mindfulness Meditation Practice, Series One*
cassette tape from www.mindfulnesstapes.com or by writing to: Stress
Reduction Tapes, PO Box 547, Lexington, MA 02420. These tapes are
narrated by Jon Kabat-Zinn, who happens to have a very soothing
voice. The tapes compliment the book, and they can be useful when
you first begin your practice because of the clear instructions
provided.

Another good resource is the CD *Meditation for Beginners* by Jack
Kornfield. This can be ordered through Amazon.com.

Cooling Products

Heat Relief Depot: (877) 879-1450 *or* www.heatreliefdepot.com

Steele Body Cooling Comfort Systems: (888) 783-3538 *or*
www.steelevest.com

There are a few programs that provide cooling products at a low cost
or free of charge, including the MS Society and the MS Association of
America (www.msaa.com).

Massage

American Massage Therapy Association (AMTA)
(312) 761-2682

Exercise

To order exercise videos of all types from Collage Video, call (800) 433-6769 or go to www.collagevideo.com

Guided Imagery

To order guided imagery tapes from Belleruth Naparstek, call (800) 800-8661. She offers a guided imagery tape called *For People with Multiple Sclerosis*. You can access Belleruth's website at: www.health journeys.com.

Biofeedback

The Association for Applied Psychophysiology and Biofeedback (800) 477-8892
Website: www.aapb.org
This organization may also be able to help you find a qualified professional in your area.

Grief Support

Grief Watch: www.griefwatch.com

On-Line Support Groups

Many people are now using the Internet to find both current information on research and treatment, as well as emotional support. The use of chat rooms and message boards is a great way for those who are unable to leave their homes or want to remain anonymous to connect with other MS patients. In addition to the resources listed here, you can find a wealth of information online by going to Google.com and searching "Multiple Sclerosis Support Groups" or simply "Multiple Sclerosis."

Thrive!: www.Thriveonline.com

The International MS Support Foundation: www.msnews.org

The National Multiple Sclerosis Society: www.nationalmssociety.org

The Multiple Sclerosis Foundation: www.msfacts.org

MSWorld: www.msworld.org

Web MD Health: Multiple Sclerosis Center: my.webmd.com/condi tion_center/mss

Adaptive Services for the Home

Adapting the Home for the Physically Challenged

A/V Health Services
P.O. Box 1622, West Sacramento CA 95691   (703) 389-4339
A videotape that shows ways to modify a home and make it more accessible.

Sentry Detection Corporation   (800) 695-0110
Provides Life Alert systems that allow you to get assistance during an emergency.

Websites Sponsored by Drug Companies

Berlex/Betaseron: www.betaseron.com

Biogen Idec/Avonex: www.avonex.com and www.MSactiveSource.com

Immunex/Novantrone: www.novantrone.com

Teva Pharmaceutical Industries/Copaxone: www.copaxone.com and www.sharedsolutions.com

Serono/Rebif: www.rebif.com

Brochures Published by the National Multiple Sclerosis Society

These can be ordered through the NMSS by calling (800) FIGHT-MS
Solving Cognitive Problems
MS and Intimacy
Plaintalk: A Booklet about MS for Families
Someone You Know Has MS: A Book for Families
When a Parent Has MS: A Teenager's Guide

Caregiver Resources

National Family Caregivers Association: www.nfcacares.org

Caregiver: www.caregiver.com

Well Spouse Foundation: www.wellspouse.org

MS World: www.msworld.org

The National Multiple Sclerosis Society: www.nationalmssociety.org

Index

⌘ ⌘ ⌘

More Hunter House Books

WOMEN LIVING WITH MULTIPLE SCLEROSIS by Judith Lynn Nichols and Her Online Group of MS Sisters

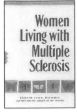

Judith Lynn Nichols was diagnosed with multiple sclerosis in 1976. Her research on the Internet eventually led to her co-founding an online group of women dedicated to supporting each other in the fight against "the MonSter."

In this book, members of the group freely discuss their experiences with MS. Some stories are painful, others are funny, many are both. Topics range from family reactions to the MS diagnosis, workplace issues, sexuality and spirituality, depression and physical pain, loss of bladder and bowel control, and assistive devices and helpful tools. Read this book, and you will feel that someone *finally* understands.

288 pages ... Paperback $14.95

LIVING *BEYOND* MULTIPLE SCLEROSIS: A Women's Guide
by Judith Lynn Nichols and Her Online Group of MS Sisters

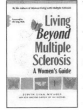

This sequel to *Women Living with Multiple Sclerosis* focuses on transcending the effects of MS. This book shares the same engaging, conversational tone as the first book. In addition to providing more time, energy, and sanity-saving techniques, this book talks about ways to live beyond the limitations MS imposes. Topics include the newest treatments for MS and how to maximize their benefits; household accessibility, safety, and remodeling; tips for choosing and using assistive devices; and how to prepare applications for Social Security Disability and insurance benefits.

288 Pages ... Paperback $14.95

GET FIT WHILE YOU SIT: Easy Workouts from Your Chair by Charlene Torkelson

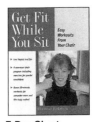

Here is a total-body workout that can be done right from your chair, anywhere. It is perfect for seniors and those with health limitations. The One-Hour Chair Program is a low-impact workout that includes light aerobics and exercises. The 5-Day Short Program features five compact workouts for those short on time.

160 pages ... Paperback $16.95 ... Spiral bound $21.95

SELF-HELP FOR HYPERVENTILATION SYNDROME: Recognizing and Correcting Your Breathing-Pattern Disorder
by Dinah Bradley

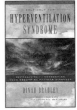

Chronic hyperventilation symptoms include breathlessness, chest pains, palpitations, broken sleep, stomach or bowel problems, dizziness, and anxiety. This book explains causes and symptoms, and presents a well-tested program that helps readers to break the hyperventilation cycle and breathe freely again.

128 pages ... Paperback $13.95 ... Third Edition

THE JOURNEY TO PAIN RELIEF: A Hands-On Guide to Breakthroughs in Pain Treatment by Phyllis Berger

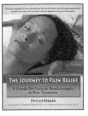

Written for pain sufferers and professionals, this book describes new techniques for blocking pain pathways with low-voltage electrical currents and acupuncture, all discussed and illustrated in detail. Other sections outline self-help options including how to increase pain-free movements with carefully selected exercises.

264 pages ... Paperback $18.95

CHRONIC FATIGUE SYNDROME, FIBROMYALGIA, AND OTHER INVISIBLE ILLNESSES:
The Comprehensive Guide
by Katrina Berne, Ph.D.

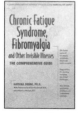

This is a definitive guide to chronic fatigue syndrome (CFS) and fibromyalgia syndrome (FMS). Both illnesses are accompanied by a puzzling mix of physical, cognitive, and emotional symptoms such as sore throat, headache, brain fog, sleep disturbances, balance problems, and depression. This book addresses what we know about the causes of CFS and FMS, and whether they are related; the wide range of symptoms and diagnostic techniques; and proven and experimental treatment and self-care options. There is a chapter on CFS and FMS in children, and invaluable advice on dealing with relationship issues and lifestyle changes.

400 pages ... Paperback $18.95 ... Third Edition

WOMEN LIVING WITH FIBROMYALGIA
by Mari Skelly with Kelley Blewster

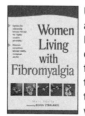

Using interviews, discussions, and personal stories, this book deals with the real-life concerns of women with fibromyalgia. Skelly highlights the strategies and therapies that a broad spectrum of women use to face FM's many challenges — from the single student pondering how FM will affect her as a woman to the mother trying to find energy to care for her family.

Topics include possible causes of FM and why it especially affects women; fifty strategies for dealing with pain, fatigue, and sleep disturbances; and exploring spirituality in the face of a disease that is difficult to diagnose and may have no cure.

320 pages ... Paperback $16.95

ALTERNATIVE TREATMENTS FOR FIBROMYALGIA AND CHRONIC FATIGUE SYNDROME: Insights from Practitioners and Patients
by Mari Skelly and Helen Walker ... Second Edition

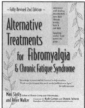

Many people suffering from FM and CFS are unable to find effective treatment and relief. This book combines personal stories from patients with interviews with practitioners of alternative therapies — including acupuncture, chiropractic, osteopathy, and reflexology; movement therapies such as tai chi, yoga, and hanna somatics; energetic healing, including reiki, thought field therapy, hypnosis, and guided imagery; and new drug combinations and guaifenesin therapy

With 40 percent new material, the new edition offers both insight into and inspiration for dealing with these challenging conditions. There are also sections on health insurance and Social Security Disability.

320 pages ... Paperback $17.95

THE ART OF GETTING WELL: A Five-Step Plan for Maximizing Health When You Have a Chronic Illness
by David Spero, R.N.

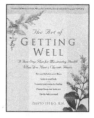

Self-management programs have become a key way for people to deal with chronic illness. In this book, David Spero offers a five-step approach to the medical, psychological, and spiritual aspects of getting well: slow down and use your energy for the things and people that matter — make small, progressive changes that build confidence — get help and nourish your social ties — value your body and treat it with affection and respect — take responsibility for getting the best care that you can.

224 pages ... Paperback $17.95

More Hunter House Books

I-CAN'T-CHEW COOKBOOK:
Delicious Soft-Diet Recipes for People with Chewing, Swallowing and Dry-Mouth Disorders *by J. Randy Wilson*

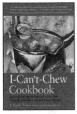

Over 40 million people in the U.S. need to eat soft foods: people with TMJ; stroke, cancer, Alzheimer's, AIDS, and lupus; and people recovering from serious surgery. This cookbook features 168 tasty and nutritious soft- or liquid-diet recipes with nutritional analyses and tips on preparation.

Endorsed by medical professionals, it contains an introductory chapter by a registered dietician and is also available in a lie-flat spiral binding.

224 pages ... Paperback $17.95 ... Spiralbound $22.95

THE JOY OF LAZINESS: Why Life is Better Slower — and How to Get There
by Peter Axt, Ph.D., and Michaela Axt-Gadermann, M.D.

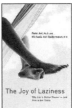

The early bird may get the worm, but late sleepers live longer! The authors — both former (and reformed) champion athletes — show why being lazy can make your immune system stronger, too much exercise can make you sick, fasting delays the aging process, and being relaxed and even-tempered makes you smarter and healthier. They also explain ways to conserve energy and monitor your stress level, and outline an exercise program that will promote both fitness and a long life.

160 pages ... Paperback $14.95

Books from the Positive Options for Health series

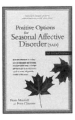

POSITIVE OPTIONS FOR SEASONAL AFFECTIVE DISORDER (SAD)
by Fiona Marshall and Peter Cheevers

About 10 million Americans suffer from SAD. This book helps distinguish the condition from classic depression and chronic fatigue, and suggests ways to alleviate the symptoms and live optimally.

144 pages ... Paperback $12.95

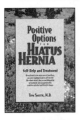

POSITIVE OPTIONS FOR HIATUS HERNIA
by Tom Smith, M.D.

A hiatus hernia is a common, potentially serious condition that occurs when the upper part of the stomach pushes through the diaphragm. This book describes tests, treatments, and self-help options.

128 pages ... Paperback $12.95

POSITIVE OPTIONS FOR ANTIPHOSPHOLIPID SYNDROME (APS)
by Triona Holden

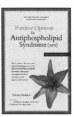

Also called Hughes syndrome and "sticky blood," APS is implicated in many serious health problems. This book identifies the symptoms and provides important information on diagnosis and treatment.

144 pages ... Paperback $12.95

POSITIVE OPTIONS FOR REFLEX SYMPATHETIC DYSTROPHY (RSD)
by Elena Juris

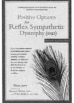

RSD, also called Complex Regional Pain Syndrome, is characterized by severe nerve pain and extreme sensitivity to touch. This detailed, sensitive book by a RSD sufferer covers medical information, practical advice, and holistic therapies.

224 pages ... Paperback $16.95

To order visit hunterhouse.com ... all prices subject to change

THE IBS HEALING PLAN: Natural Ways to Beat Your Symptoms
by Theresa Cheung

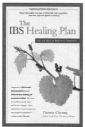

Irritable bowel syndrome (IBS) affects 15–20 percent of adults in the U.S. Written to help those suffering from the abdominal pain, bloating, and irregular bowel habits that accompany IBS, this book focuses on five key areas: diet, supplements, complementary therapies, stress management, and working with your doctor. Also covers natural remedies including acupuncture, supplements, and dietary changes, and the benefits and drawbacks of over-the-counter and prescription drugs.

168 pages ... 9 illus. ... Paperback $14.95

THE ANTI-INFLAMMATION DIET & RECIPE BOOK: Protect Yourself and Your Family from Heart Disease, Arthritis, Diabetes, Allergies — and More
by Jessica K. Black, N.D.

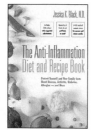

Inflammation is linked to chronic illnesses like heart disease and arthritis. Anti-inflammation diets emphasize whole foods, reducing processed sugars, more vegetables to promote simpler and easier digestion, and avoiding foods with pesticides and hormones.

Jessica Black discusses the science behind anti-inflammation diets then gives . 125 recipes, most of which can be prepared quickly and easily at home. Each recipe includes a healthy ingredient tip, substitution suggestions, and a complete nutritional analysis. There are sample menus for summer and winter, as well as a substitutions chart for modifying recipes to increase their healing potential.

256 pages ... 4 illus. ... 14 charts ... 5 tables ... 125 recipes ... Paperback $16.95 ... Spiralbound $19.95

THE ULTIMATE METABOLISM DIET: Eat Right for Your Metabolic Type by Scott Rigden, MD, with Barbara Schiltz, RN

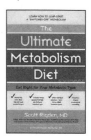

This book uses quizzes and questionnaires to help readers determine which of the five major metabolic disorders they are affected by: carbohydrate sensitivity, metabolic syndrome, food hypersensitivities, functional hormonal imbalance, or impaired liver detoxification.

For each disorder, Dr. Rigden provides specific diet, exercise, supplement, and OTC drug-related suggestions that are designed to work with the body's strengths and weaknesses. He includes a chapter on emotional eating, as well as case studies, charts, recipes, and descriptions of techniques that have been highly effective at his clinic in Arizona. The recommendations are based on highly successful practice and extensive research.

264 pages ... 30 charts | 22 recipes ... Paperback $15.95

WOMEN'S SEXUAL PASSAGES: Finding Pleasure and Intimacy at Every Stage of Life by Elizabeth Davis

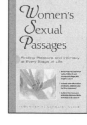

Davis explores the mystery of how and why women's desire changes in the course of a lifetime under the influence of biological rhythms, hormones, pregnancy, cultural attitudes, menopause, and aging.

To help women truly understand their sexuality she looks at the effects of stress, overwork, major life events, relationship upheaval, and sexual abuse. New chapters address sexual awakening and sex in the later years, and how hormonal changes at menopause are linked to increased insight and assertiveness.

288 pages ... 1 illus. ... Paperback $15.95